TOP TRAILS™

California Central Coast

Written by

Brian Milne

 WILDERNESS PRESS · BERKELEY, CALIFORNIA

To Payton, my new hiking buddy

Top Trails California Central Coast

1st EDITION May 2008

Copyright © 2008 by Brian Milne

All photos copyright by Brian Milne, except where noted
Maps: Lohnes + Wright
Cover design: Frances Baca Design and Lisa Pletka
Interior design: Frances Baca Design
Book production: Larry B. Van Dyke
Book editor: Elaine Merrill

ISBN: 978-0-89997-437-8
UPC: 7-19609-97437-6

Manufactured in Canada

Published by: **Wilderness Press**
               1345 8th Street
               Berkeley, CA 94710
               (800) 443-7227; FAX (510) 558-1696
               info@wildernesspress.com
               www.wildernesspress.com
Visit our website for a complete listing of our books and for ordering information.

Cover photos: View from atop Cerro Cabrillo above Morro Bay, by Brian Milne;
              great white heron (inset), by Brian Milne

SAFETY NOTICE: Although Wilderness Press and the author have made every attempt to ensure that the information in this book is accurate at press time, they are not responsible for any loss, damage, injury, or inconvenience that may occur to anyone while using this book. You are responsible for your own safety and health while in the wilderness. The fact that a trail is described in this book does not mean that it will be safe for you. Be aware that trail conditions can change from day to day. Always check local conditions and know your own limitations.

The Top Trails™ Series

Wilderness Press

When Wilderness Press published *Sierra North* in 1967, no other trail guide like it existed for the Sierra backcountry. The first print run sold out in less than two months and its success heralded the beginning of Wilderness Press. Since we were founded more than 40 years ago, we have expanded our territories to cover California, Alaska, Hawaii, the U.S. Southwest, the Pacific Northwest, New England, Canada, and Baja California.

Wilderness Press continues to publish comprehensive, accurate, and readable outdoor books. Hikers, backpackers, kayakers, skiers, snowshoers, climbers, cyclists, and trail runners rely on Wilderness Press for accurate outdoor adventure information.

Top Trails

In its Top Trails guides, Wilderness Press has paid special attention to organization so that you can find the perfect hike each and every time. Whether you're looking for a steep trail to test yourself on or a walk in the park, a romantic waterfall or a city view, Top Trails will lead you there.

Each Top Trails guide contains trails for everyone. The trails selected provide a sampling of the best that the region has to offer. These are the "must-do" hikes, walks, runs, and bike rides, with every feature of the area represented.

Every book in the Top Trails series offers:

- The Wilderness Press commitment to accuracy and reliability
- Ratings and rankings for each trail
- Distances and approximate times
- Easy-to-follow trail notes
- Maps and permit information

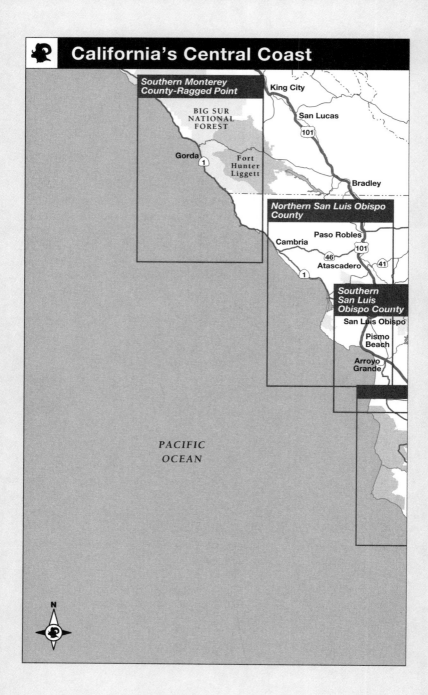

California's Central Coast

Southern Monterey County-Ragged Point

King City

BIG SUR NATIONAL FOREST

San Lucas

101

Gorda 1

Fort Hunter Liggett

Bradley

Northern San Luis Obispo County

Paso Robles

Cambria

101

46

Atascadero

41

1

Southern San Luis Obispo County

San Luis Obispo

Pismo Beach

Arroyo Grande

PACIFIC OCEAN

N

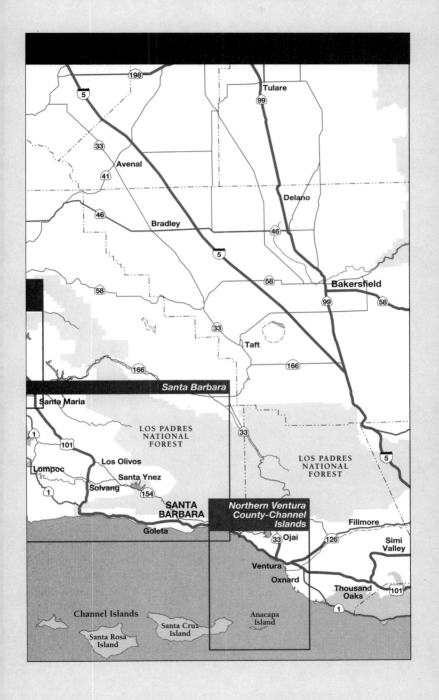

California Central Coast Trails

Trail Number and Name	Page	Difficulty -12345+	Length in Miles	Type	Hiking	Horses	Running	Biking	Child Friendly	Handicap Access	Fee
1. Southern Monterey County — Ragged Point											
1 McWay Falls	29	1	0.6	Out & Back	Hiking				Child Friendly	Handicap Access	
2 Cone Peak	33	5	4.5	Out & Back	Hiking		Running				
3 Limekiln Creek	39	3	2.1	Out & Back	Hiking		Running				$
4 Jade Cove	45	3	1.5	Loop	Hiking		Running		Child Friendly		
5 Salmon Creek Falls	51	4	6.4	Out & Back	Hiking		Running				
6 Ragged Point Nature Trail	55	4	1.0	Out & Back	Hiking						
7 San Carpoforo Creek	61	2	1.4	Out & Back	Hiking		Running		Child Friendly		
2. Northern San Luis Obispo County											
8 San Simeon Point	79	3	2.5	Out & Back	Hiking		Running		Child Friendly		
9 Villa Creek	83	2	2.4	Out & Back	Hiking		Running				
10 Cerro Cabrillo	87	4	2.5	Out & Back	Hiking	Horses	Running	Biking			
11 Elfin Forest	93	1	1.0	Loop	Hiking	Horses	Running	Biking	Child Friendly	Handicap Access	
12 Montaña de Oro Bluff Trail	97	2	3.3	Out & Back	Hiking		Running	Biking	Child Friendly		
13 Coon Creek	103	3	4.4	Out & Back	Hiking		Running				
14 Cerro Alto	109	4	4.0	Out & Back	Hiking	Horses	Running	Biking			$
15 Jim Green Trail	113	2	1.7	Loop	Hiking	Horses	Running	Biking	Child Friendly		
16 Rinconada	117	4	4.6	Loop	Hiking	Horses	Running	Biking			
17 Blinn Ranch Trail	123	5	18	Out & Back	Hiking	Horses	Running	Biking			$
18 Salinas River Parkway	129	2	2.2	Out & Back	Hiking		Running	Biking	Child Friendly	Handicap Access	
3. Southern San Luis Obispo County											
19 West Cuesta Ridge	145	4	10	Out & Back	Hiking	Horses	Running	Biking			
20 Eagle Rock	149	3	1.8	Out & Back	Hiking		Running				$
21 Bishop Peak	155	4	3.0	Out & Back	Hiking		Running				

Legend

USES & ACCESS
- Hiking
- Horses
- Running
- Biking
- Child Friendly
- Handicap Access
- $ Fee
- Permit Required
- Dogs Allowed

TYPE
- Loop
- Out & Back
- Point-to-Point

DIFFICULTY
-12345+
less   more

TERRAIN
- River or Stream
- Waterfall
- Lake
- Beach
- Tide Pools
- Canyon
- Mountain

FLORA & FAUNA
- Wildflowers
- Fall Color
- Birds
- Wildlife

FEATURES
- Historic Interest
- Geologic Interest
- Great Views
- Steep
- Secluded
- Camping

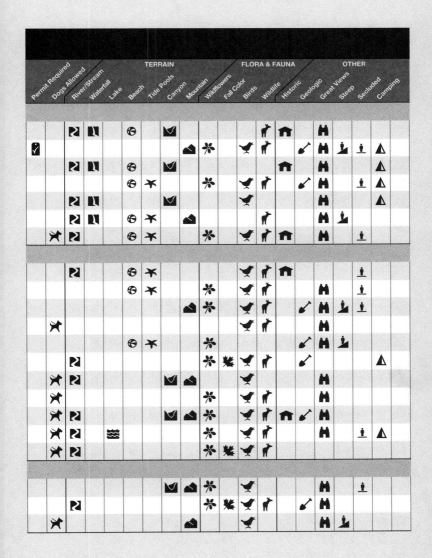

California Central Coast Trails

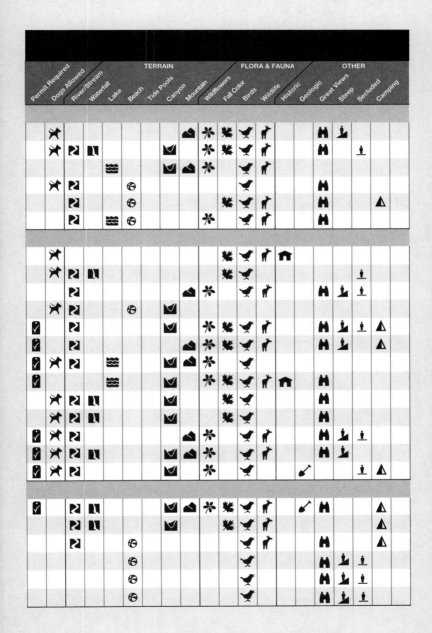

Contents

Using Top Trails™

Organization of Top Trails

Top Trails is designed to make identifying the perfect trail easy and enjoyable, and to make every outing a success and a pleasure. With this book you'll find it's a snap to find the right trail, whether you're planning a major hike or just a sociable stroll with friends.

The Region

Top Trails begins with the **California Central Coast Regional Map** (pages iv-v), displaying the entire region covered by the guide and providing a geographic overview. The map is clearly marked to show which area is covered by each chapter.

After the regional map comes the **California Central Coast Trails Table** (pages vi-ix), which lists every trail covered in the guide, along with

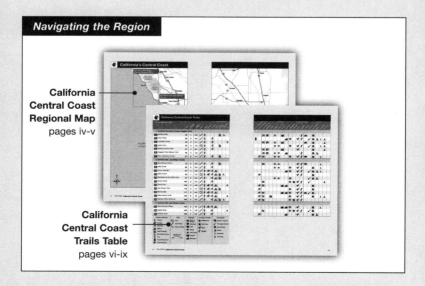

Navigating the Region

California Central Coast Regional Map pages iv-v

California Central Coast Trails Table pages vi-ix

attributes for each trail. A quick reading of the regional map and the trails table will give you a good overview of the entire region covered by the book.

The Areas

The region covered in each book is divided into areas, with each chapter corresponding to one area in the region.

Each area chapter starts with information to help you choose and enjoy a trail every time out. Use the table of contents or the regional map to identify an area of interest, then turn to the area chapter to find the following:

- An overview of the area, including park and permit information
- An area map with all trails clearly marked
- A trail feature table providing trail-by-trail details
- Trail summaries, written in a lively, accessible style

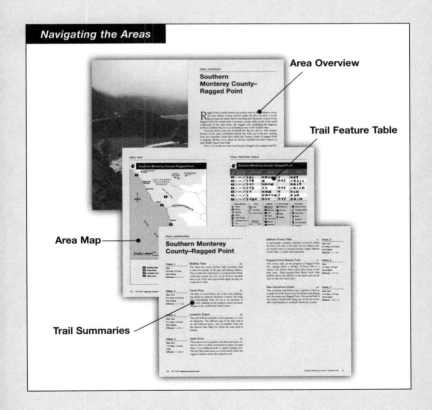

Navigating the Areas

Area Overview

Trail Feature Table

Area Map

Trail Summaries

The Trails

The basic building block of the Top Trails guide is the trail entry. Each one is arranged to make finding and following the trail as simple as possible, with all pertinent information presented in this easy-to-follow format:

- A trail map
- Trail descriptors covering difficulty, length, and other essential data
- A written trail description
- Trail milestones providing easy-to follow, turn-by-turn trail directions

Some trail descriptions offer additional information:

- An elevation profile
- Trail options
- Trail highlights

In the margins of the trail entries, keep your eyes open for graphic icons that signal passages in the text.

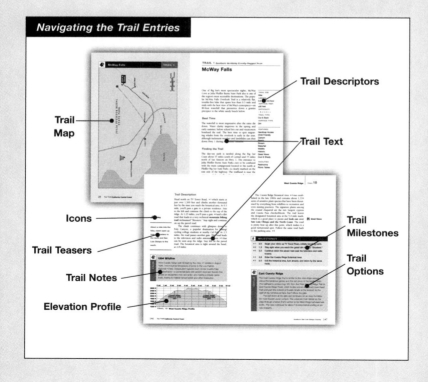

Choosing a Trail

Top Trails provides several different ways of choosing a trail, all presented in easy-to-read tables, charts, and maps.

Location

If you know in general where you want to go, Top Trails makes it easy to find the right trail in the right place. Each chapter begins with a large-scale map showing the starting point of every trail in that area.

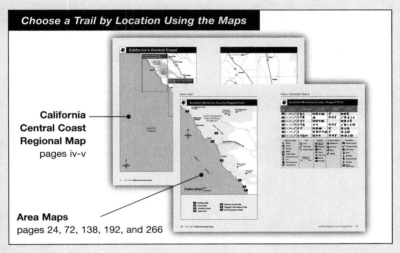

Choose a Trail by Location Using the Maps

California Central Coast Regional Map
pages iv-v

Area Maps
pages 24, 72, 138, 192, and 266

Features

This guide describes the top trails of the California Central Coast region. Each trail is chosen because it offers one or more features that make it interesting. Using the trail descriptors, summaries, and tables, you can quickly examine all the trails for the features they offer, or seek a particular feature among the list of trails.

Season and Condition

Time of year and current conditions can be important factors in selecting the best trail. For example, an exposed grassland trail may be a riot of color in early spring, but an oven-baked taste of hell in midsummer. Wherever relevant, Top Trails identifies the best and worst conditions for the trails you plan to hike.

Difficulty

Each trail has an overall difficulty rating on a scale of 1 to 5, which takes into consideration length, elevation change, exposure, trail quality, and more, to create one (admittedly subjective) rating.

The ratings assume you are an able-bodied adult in reasonably good shape using the trail for hiking. The ratings also assume normal weather conditions—clear and dry.

Readers should make an honest assessment of their own abilities and adjust time estimates accordingly. Also, rain, snow, heat, and poor visibility can all affect the pace on even the easiest of trails.

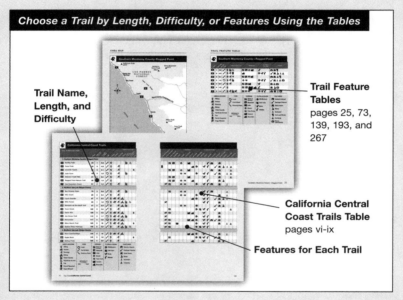

Choose a Trail by Length, Difficulty, or Features Using the Tables

Trail Name, Length, and Difficulty

Trail Feature Tables
pages 25, 73, 139, 193, and 267

California Central Coast Trails Table
pages vi–ix

Features for Each Trail

Vertical Feet

This important measurement is often underestimated by hikers and bikers when gauging the difficulty of a trail. The Top Trails measurement accounts for all elevation change, not simply the difference between the highest and lowest points, so that rolling terrain with lots of ups and downs, will be identifiable.

The calculation of vertical feet in the Top Trails series is accomplished by a combination of trail measurement and computer-aided estimation. For routes that begin and end at the same spot—i.e., loop or out and back—the vertical gain exactly matches the vertical descent. With a point-to-point route, the vertical gain and loss will most likely differ, and both figures will be provided in the text.

Finally, some of trail entries in the Top Trails series have an elevation profile, an easy means for visualizing the topography of the route. These profiles graphically depict the elevation throughout the length of the trail.

 Top Trails Difficulty Ratings

1 A short trail, generally level, which can be completed in one hour or less.

2 A route of 1 to 3 miles, with some up and down, which can be completed in one to two hours.

3 A longer route, up to 5 miles, with uphill and/or downhill sections.

4 A long or steep route, perhaps more than 5 miles, or with climbs of more than 1,000 vertical feet.

5 The most severe route, both long and steep, more than 5 miles long, with climbs of more than 1,000 vertical feet.

Surface Type

Each trail entry provides information about the surface of the trail. This is useful in determining what type of footwear or bicycle is appropriate. Surface type should also be considered when checking the weather—on a rainy day a dirt surface can be a muddy slog; an asphalt surface might be a better choice (although asphalt can be slick when wet).

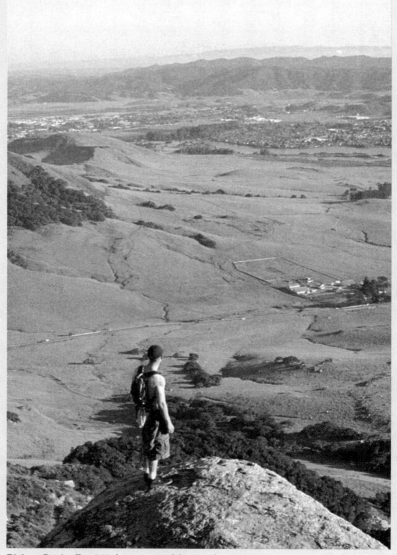

Bishop Peak *offers 360-degree views of the city of San Luis Obispo.*

Introduction to the California Central Coast

Everyone knows about the never-ending recreational activities in Southern California, and the breathtaking hikes around Big Sur to the north, but little has been made of the outdoor opportunities in between, where countless trails keep hikers, mountain bikers, and equestrians happy all year long.

The Central Coast of California is truly a hidden treasure, buried halfway between San Francisco and Los Angeles. With miles of unspoiled beaches, poppy-dotted fields, precious mountain peaks, burbling streams, and gin-clear lakes, along with other natural escapes, the "Middle Kingdom" is the perfect destination for those looking to flee the rigors of everyday life. And the best part about these trails is that they see very few crowds, tucked away as they are in small-town communities within Monterey, San Luis Obispo, Santa Barbara, and Ventura counties.

Top Trails California Central Coast will take you through the best trails this region has to offer. Whether it's an easy stroll to the majestic pools of Salmon Creek Falls, or an 18-mile trek around the perimeter of Santa Margarita Lake, this book has a special getaway for everyone to discover.

Geography

For the purpose of this book, the Central Coast region encompasses at least a portion of four counties—Monterey, San Luis Obispo, Santa Barbara, and Ventura—and includes a wide variety of geographical and ecological conditions.

This guide focuses on hikes in the Central Coast portion of the Los Padres National Forrest, the volcanic plugs and North Coast preserves in San Luis Obispo County, the sprawling single tracks in the Santa Barbara foothills and Santa Ynez Recreation Areas, and the southern portion of the Big Sur coastline and Salinas River Valley. Additionally, there are a couple of must-see hikes in Northern Ventura County, along with a handful of Channel Islands getaways.

The northern portion of the Central Coast region is defined by its rugged coastline, which eventually gives way to the Estero Bay to the south and the estuary at Morro Bay. The ragged Pacific coastline fades into dune and beach environments south of the Diablo Canyon coastline. The beach community winds down to another significant wetland located at the mouth of the Santa Clara River.

The San Andreas Fault shapes the geography, with a majority of the mountain ranges running parallel to the coast in a north-south direction. Over time, valleys have been formed as a result of the two continental plates colliding along the fault line. The chain of volcanic plugs in San Luis Obispo County is referred to as the "Nine Sisters" (however, three of the plugs are closed to hiking). The peaks were formed more than 20 million years ago as part of the Franciscan Formation, spanning from Morro Rock in Morro Bay to Islay Hill in San Luis Obispo.

The primary mountain range in Monterey and San Luis Obispo counties is the Santa Lucia Mountains, while the Santa Ynez Mountains stretch to the south, separating the inland and coastal communities of Santa Barbara County.

Flora

The Central Coast has a wide variety of plant communities, which are detailed throughout the trail descriptions. Coastal scrub dominates the coast, providing an ever-present buffer between the ocean and the rolling foothills that define the region. Common shrubs along the coastal bluffs include coyote brush, lilac, and various fragrant shrubs and herbs like sagebrush and hedge nettle. In the spring, the lupine, sticky monkey flower, and other wildflowers help mix in some color along the coast.

The chaparral community typically covers the driest slopes and makes for tough hiking conditions because the waist-high brush rarely offers refuge from the sun. Manzanita and other brush species make up a majority of the vegetation. Yucca stands out in this environment in the spring and early summer because of its tall stalk and white flowers. The purple wild hyacinth and pink dudleya add color to the golden brown hillsides in the summer.

Grassland can be found alongside the coastal scrub and within the dry interior around tree-studded foothills and thickets of chaparral. This is where the state flower, the California poppy, flourishes along with colorful lupines and shooting stars in the spring.

Hikers searching for a reprieve from the summer heat need look no farther than the oak woodland. The Los Padres National Forest is made up of miles and miles of woodland sheltered by blue, valley, and coast live oaks.

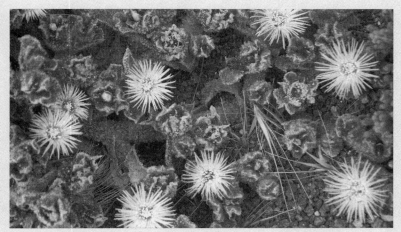

Santa Cruz Island *is home to spectacular wildflower displays in the spring.*

The mixed evergreen forest shelters many of the same animal species as the oak woodland, but is found at higher, rockier elevations. The forest includes everything from the Santa Lucia fir to the ponderosa and sugar pine.

Fauna

Because the Central Coast is along the Pacific flyway, it contains more than 80 noteworthy birding sites along the Central Coast Birding Trail, and eight Globally Important Bird Areas as recognized by the American Bird Conservancy. Christmas bird counts in Morro Bay, one of the best birding destinations in the country, have numbered above the 200-species mark.

The most recognizable birds along the coastline include the endangered brown pelican, the threatened western snowy plover, and the delisted peregrine falcon. The falcons can be seen nesting on the north side of Morro Rock in Morro Bay.

Other birds of prey on the Central Coast include turkey vultures, northern harriers, and a half dozen species of hawks. The red-tailed hawk is the most common hawk in the area, although red-shouldered hawks and sharp-shinned hawks also are often seen. An occasional California condor or bald eagle also can be spotted in the Los Padres National Forest, although sightings are rare outside the main lookouts in the area.

If the birds along the Central Coast are the top attraction, the marine mammals are a close second.

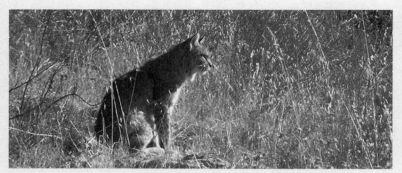

Bobcats are common *around the perimeter of Santa Margarita Lake.*

From December through April, this section of the California coastline is ideal for viewing gray whales. Humpback whales also are common up and down the coast and can be seen on clear days from region's many bluff-top trails. In northern San Luis Obispo County, just north of Hearst Castle, the northern elephant seal can be seen at the Piedras Blancas rookery. Winter is the peak viewing season for elephant seals, which stack up on the beach by the hundreds. Other marine mammals in this region include porpoises, harbor seals, sea lions, and sea otters.

The Central Coast also is home to one of the largest monarch butterfly groves in the country. From October to February, 100,000 butterflies migrate to the eucalyptus grove at Pismo State Beach. Farther inland, the butterflies do not congregate in such unusually large colonies; their typical numbers are the same as you'd find in any other area of the state.

With a population in the thousands, mule deer are the most common and probably the largest mammals you'll see in oak woodland areas. The occasional black bear or mountain lion is sighted on backcountry trails, although encounters are rare. Nevertheless, trail users are encouraged to hike with a partner on remote trails.

Coyotes and bobcats are much more common in this area, although they pose no danger unless cornered or harassed. They are often seen streaking across backcountry roads or scampering down canyon trails in search of food.

Other common mammals include foxes, raccoons, rabbits, squirrels, wood rats, and mice.

Many reptiles also can be found along the inland and ridgetop trails, including various lizards and snakes. Rattlesnakes are far more common in the area than mountain lions or bears, so be wary when hiking in grassland or chaparral-covered trails.

The seasonal streams in the area are home to rainbow trout, wild steelhead, and various frogs, salamanders, and turtles.

When to Go

There really isn't a bad time to hike on the Central Coast.

Because most of the trails in this book are close to the ocean, the mild coastal temperatures make for picture-perfect hiking conditions throughout much of the year.

Along the coast, the only weather worry hikers have is the gloomy marine layer. Hiking in breathable, layered clothing can help fend off the wind and moisture that come with beach and bluff-top hikes.

Trails along the Central Coast's interior are where the conditions become a little more extreme. The inland valleys can endure freezing temperatures in the winter, although things usually warm up enough for a hike in the afternoon. Snow is extremely rare this side of the Sierra Nevada, although the Figueroa Mountain Recreation Area sees occasional snowfall when large winter storms come through.

The rainy season typically runs from October to March, although the Central Coast is lucky to see 15 inches of rain each year. When it does rain, many forest roads leading to the more remote hikes are closed or become impassable for small cars.

In the summertime, peak and ridgeline trails can see triple-digit temperatures, so be sure to bring plenty of water on those hikes when it's warm. Avoid the dog days of summer by sticking to morning and evening hikes or afternoon hikes on trails with plenty of tree cover.

While the weather and air quality aren't usually factors on the Central Coast, many hikers swear March and May are the best times to hike because of the fantastic wildflower displays sprinkled about the vibrant green hillsides. Popular wildflowers in the area include shooting stars, California poppies, lupines, and Mariposa lilies. By June, many of the barren inland hillsides have turned dry and golden brown. The spring also is a good time for all the waterfall and streamside hikes, as stream flows are usually at their highest levels.

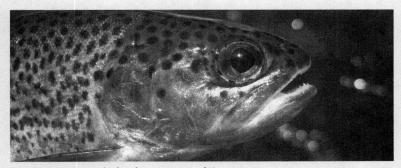

Steelhead trout *can be found in many Central Coast streams.*

Trail Selection

Three criteria were used in selecting the trails for this guide. First, the signature hikes, peak climbs, trail runs, and/or mountain-bike trails that define the region were included. Second, trails that capture the diversity of the Central Coast's trail system were included to balance out the book and provide both coastal and inland hiking opportunities. Instead of stacking up all of the hikes in Montaña de Oro, Big Sur, or in the Santa Barbara foothills, this guide strives to present hikers with a better variety of trails, and includes many tracks that aren't found in other guides.

Third, convenience was a major factor. Most of the trails on the Central Coast are quick, painless hikes that can be tackled before work, during a lunch break, or after work before the sun disappears into the Pacific. As a bonus, nearly all of the hikes are accessible via U.S. Hwy. 101 or highways 1 and 154, which makes each of them a feasible day trip.

Key Features

Top Trails books contain information about "features" for each trail. Even though the Central Coast is a relatively small slice of California's golden coast, the region is blessed with a wide diversity of terrain.

Water lovers and anglers have plenty of lakes and beach hikes, while climbers have many peaks to keep them busy. Add an interesting mixture of open-meadows hikes and streamside treks through the Los Padres National Forest, and there's a trail here on the Central Coast for just about everyone.

Multiple Uses

All the trails described in this guide are suitable for hiking. Because many of the trails are relatively short hikes, they also are popular for jogging. Santa Barbara and San Luis Obispo counties also have made a conscious effort to provide mountain bikers, equestrians, and dog walkers with plenty of options as well. It is worth noting, however, that many of the state park trails prohibit dogs, horses, and mountain bikes.

Trail Safety

There aren't many hazards to worry about while hiking on the Central Coast, although trail users should always remain cautious of ticks, rattlesnakes, and poison oak. In recent years, there also have been a few mountain lion sightings, particularly in San Luis Obispo County, although confrontations are extremely rare.

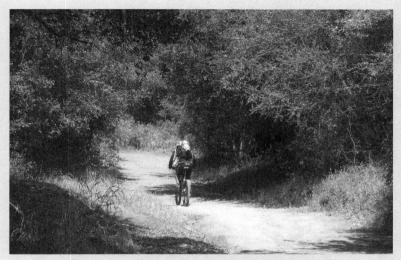

A mountain biker *starts his climb toward Inspiration Point.*

Ticks can be found on just about every hike in this guide, especially in the late spring and early summer. The best way to prevent bites is to use repellant and check your clothing and body frequently for the small black and red arachnids. The same rule of thumb should be used for dogs, which often get ticks behind their ears and upper legs. Tick collars and flea or tick treatment drops can help keep ticks and fleas away from your pooch.

Rattlesnakes are common at the drier elevations and on many of the inland hikes in San Luis Obispo, Santa Barbara, and Ventura counties. Rattlesnakes often prefer rocky areas, so climb with caution when rock hopping or ascending the many peaks on the Central Coast.

Poison oak seems to prefer the shady canyons and streamside trails along the coast. The plant can be identified by its distinctive three-leafed structure. Avoid contact with poison oak at all cost and be sure to immediately wash any clothing that may have brushed up against it.

Mountain lion sightings will likely increase in the future thanks to urban sprawl. While confrontations with predators like mountain lions or bears are still very rare, it's worth heeding the following advice:

- Avoid hiking alone.
- Keep children at your side and dogs on a leash.
- Never turn your back or run from a predator. Instead, throw your hands in their air and try to make yourself look as large as possible. Shouting or blowing a whistle may help drive predators away. Use rocks and sticks to defend yourself if attacked.

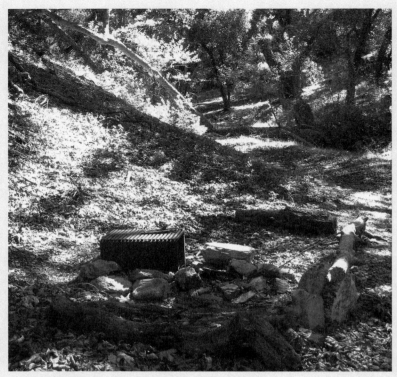

An Adventure Pass *is needed to backpack to Ballard Camp.*

Camping and Permits

There are a number of campgrounds on the coast and along the shores of the inland lakes in this area. There also are dozens of camping sites in the Los Padres National Forest, including hike-in sites along with developed camping areas.

The most popular campgrounds, along the coast at state parks and beaches, fill up quickly in the summer. Many of these campgrounds are available on a first-come basis, although some sites allow reservations through www.ReserveAmerica.com.

Trail users should note that hikes in the Los Padres National Forest often require a National Forest Adventure Pass, although the program is being phased out in some areas. An Adventure Pass can be purchased at ranger stations and sporting goods retailers, including Big 5 in San Luis Obispo and Santa Barbara. The $30 passes can be ordered by calling (909) 382-2622.

Note from the Author

From 2006 to 2007 I hiked, and often re-hiked, every trail listed in this guide. Along the way, I suffered a stress fracture in my foot (I had never before broken a bone in my body), contacted poison oak for the first time, and lost my wife's $300 digital camera on a hike up to Inspiration Point in Santa Barbara. I learned firsthand that hiking in the backcountry, or on boardwalk trails along the beach for that matter, can take a toll on the body and your gear—so always remember to hike with caution and to be prepared for the unexpected.

Keep in mind that the trails listed in this guide are constantly evolving, thanks to the efforts of county and city governments, along with the work of dozens of conservation-minded organizations in the area.

It also is important to note that different maps and GPS units will offer slight variations in trail routes and distances. While researching this guide, I used a Garmin eTrex Legend and MapSource software to export the maps. While I have made every effort to include accurate trail conditions and logistical details, some descriptions will likely change with time as hikes are improved or degraded. I hope this guide will help the next generation of hikers appreciate these trails and prevent the latter from occurring so that everyone can continue to enjoy all of the amazing outdoor opportunities this region has to offer.

More to Come Thanks to the many conservation and trail-improvement groups in the area, the land and trails that make this region special are being protected and preserved throughout the entire Central Coast area. Land acquisitions continue to open up private lands. Even as the final touches were being made on this guide, there were a handful of new trails in the works.

Among the proposed trails are the following:

- A 3.0-mile trek to coastal lands north of the Diablo Canyon nuclear power plant was under development—a bluff-top trail that runs from the southern boundary of Montaña de Oro State Park to Crowbar Canyon. The trail would open a section of coastline that was closed for years because of security concerns. Shortly before this book went to press, a 1.0-mile loop to Point Buchon had already been opened to the public. The trailhead for this hike is at the parking area for the Coon Creek Trail (Trail 13 in this guide).
- Because of public demand, the San Luis Obispo County Parks and Recreation Commission was reworking its trail plans for the first time in nearly 38 years, which could bring a handful of new trails and bicycle routes to the area.

- The California Conservation Corps recently carved a 6.0-mile trail out of the unspoiled terrain behind Santa Margarita Lake. The trail will be accessible off the 18-mile Blinn Ranch Trail (Trail 17 in this guide).
- The newly finished Fiscalini Ranch bluff and Moonstone Dr. trails in Cambria have made it easier for users of all ages to enjoy hiking. A Marine Terrace trail also was in the works.
- Multiple trails have been proposed in San Luis Obispo and Monterey counties as part of the Upper Salinas River Corridor Enhancement Project. Working trails into the system would provide long-awaited access to the Salinas River and allow conservation groups to add plant life that would reduce erosion and improve the river's mostly nonexistent flows for much of the year.
- The most significant move for trail enhancement came in 2004, when California State Parks acquired 959 acres and 13 miles of coastline as part of a $95 million Hearst Ranch conservation deal. The historic acquisition provides access to the golden coastline that parallels U.S. Hwy. 1 up to Big Sur.

Note about the 2008 Proposed Park Closures

In 2008, California Governor Arnold Schwarzenegger proposed closing or partially closing nearly 50 California state parks, including some popular parks covered in this guide. As of press time, the possibility of park closures was unclear.

The trips potentially affected include Trail 3, Trail 8, Trail 9, Trail 12, Trail 13, and Trail 28.

For more information about the current status of these parks, call California State Parks at 800-777-0369 or visit www.parks. ca.gov.

On the Trail

Every outing should begin with proper preparation, which usually takes just minutes. Even the easiest trail can turn up unexpected surprises. Hikers never think that they will get lost or suffer an injury, but accidents do happen. Simple precautions can make the difference between a good story and a dangerous situation.

Use the Top Trails ratings and descriptions to determine if a particular trail is a good match with your fitness and energy level, given current conditions and time of year. Pay particular attention to the **Best Time** description given for each trail.

Have a Plan

Choose Wisely The first step to enjoying any trail is to match the trail to your abilities. It's no use overestimating your experience or fitness—know your abilities and limitations, and use the **Top Trails Difficulty Rating** that accompanies each trail.

Leave Word The most basic of precautions is leaving word of your intentions with family or friends. Many people will hike the backcountry their entire lives without ever relying on this safety net, but establishing this simple habit is free insurance.

It's best to leave specific information—location, trail name, intended time of travel—with a responsible person. However, if this is not possible or if plans change at the last minute, you should still leave word. If there is a registration process available, make use of it. If there is a ranger station or park office, check in.

Review the Route Before embarking on any trail, be sure to read the entire description and study the map. It isn't necessary to memorize every detail, but it is worthwhile to have a clear mental picture of the trail and the general area.

If the trail and terrain are complex, augment the trail guide with a topographic map; Top Trails will point out when this could be useful. Maps as well as current weather and trail condition information are often available from local ranger and park stations.

Check Before Going It's a good idea to check in with the local ranger or land management agency to determine the status of the trail and the roads to the trailhead, particularly just after a storm. Roads and trails may be washed out by floods.

Prep and Plan

- Know your abilities and your limitations.
- Leave word about your plans.
- Know the area and the route.

Carry the Essentials

Proper preparation for any type of trail use includes gathering certain essential items to carry. Trip checklists will vary tremendously by trail and conditions.

Clothing When the weather is good, light, comfortable clothing is the obvious choice. It's easy to believe that very little spare clothing is needed, but a prepared hiker has something tucked away for any emergency from a surprise shower to an unexpected overnight stay in a remote area.

Clothing includes proper footwear, essential for hiking and running trails. As a trail becomes more demanding, you will need footwear that performs. Running shoes are fine for many trails. If you will be carrying substantial weight or encountering sustained rugged terrain, step up to hiking boots.

In hot, sunny weather, proper clothing includes a hat, sunglasses, long-sleeved shirt and sunscreen. In cooler weather, particularly when it's wet, carry waterproof outer garments and quick-drying undergarments (avoid cotton). As general rule, whatever the conditions, bring layers that can be combined or removed to provide comfort and protection from the elements in a wide variety of conditions.

Also, long pants and long-sleeved shirts are a useful first line of defense against poison oak, ticks, and mosquitoes.

Water Never embark on a trail without carrying water. At all times, particularly in warm weather, adequate water is of key importance. Experts recommend at least 2 quarts of water per day, and when hiking in heat a gallon or more may be more appropriate. At the extreme, dehydration can be life threatening. More commonly, inadequate water brings fatigue and muscle aches.

For most outings, unless the day is very hot or the trail very long, you should plan to carry sufficient water for the entire trail. Unfortunately, natural water sources are usually questionable, and may be contaminated with bacteria, viruses, and other pollutants.

Water Treatment If it's necessary to make use of trailside water, you should filter or treat it. There are three methods for treating water: boiling, chemical treatment, and filtering. Boiling is best, but often impractical—it requires a heat source, a pot, and time. Chemical treatments, available in sporting goods stores, handle some problems, including the troublesome giardia parasite, but will not combat many chemical pollutants. The preferred method is filtration, which removes giardia and other contaminants and doesn't leave any unpleasant aftertaste.

If this hasn't convinced you to carry all the water you need, one final admonishment: Be prepared for surprises. Water sources described in the text or on maps can change course or dry up completely. Never run your water bottle dry in expectation of the next source; fill up when water is available and always keep a little in reserve.

 Food

While not as critical as water, food is energy and its importance shouldn't be underestimated. Avoid foods that are hard to digest, such as candy bars and potato chips. Carry high-energy, fast-digesting foods: nutrition bars, dehydrated fruit, gorp, jerky. Bring a little extra food—it's good protection against an outing that turns unexpectedly long, perhaps due to weather or losing your way.

Pests and Hazards

As much as we like to think of the outdoors as our home, it can surprise us with some annoyances and pests like poison oak, ticks, mosquitoes, and rattlesnakes.

A number of the trails may support thickets of trailside poison oak. People susceptible to poison oak should wear long pants and long-sleeved shirts to avoid poison oak rash. If you suspect that poison oak has touched your skin, rinse off in a nearby stream or lake and be sure to shower as soon as you get home. Consult your doctor about treatments to help you avoid and heal from poison oak rash.

Trails may also harbor ticks lurking in the trailside vegetation. As a precaution against Lyme disease, which is spread by ticks, it is a good idea to avoid getting a tick bite by wearing a long-sleeved shirt. Tuck your pant legs into your boots. Check your appendages frequently for ticks. Wear light-colored clothing to spot ticks more easily. If you are bitten by a tick, clutch it firmly between two fingers and pull it out. Even though most ticks are not disease carriers, it is best to save the tick in a baggie or film canister. If your tick bite becomes inflamed, acquires a suspicious bulls-eye-like ring around it, or if you come down soon after the bite with flu-like symptoms, consult you doctor immediately and be sure to bring the tick for identification. The long-term affects of Lyme disease can be both permanent and debilitating.

Depending on the time of the year, you may encounter mosquitoes, which can, in rare instances, carry encephalitis or the West Nile virus. But typically, you simply have to be concerned about the obnoxious itching bite of these pests. Again, a long-sleeved shirt is a good first line of defense, along with mosquito repellent.

Rattlesnakes are common on many of the Central Coast trails. Despite these snakes' bad rap, rattlesnake bites are rare in California, and rattlers and other snakes perform an important ecosystem function by eating rats, mice, and other small mammals that would soon strip most of the vegetation from our outdoor areas if they were not kept in check. Snakes are cold-blooded and may be found in the middle of a trail or in other open spaces sunning themselves. Just be sure to look ahead of you as you walk along a trail and be alert for the telltale rattling. Be sure to look on the other side before stepping over or sitting on logs and rocks. Rattlesnakes want nothing more than to be left alone, so avoid harassing, following, or poking at a rattler.

Attacks by mountain lions and bears on humans are very rare in California. The smaller and usually non-aggressive California black bear is more of a threat to your camping food than to anything else.

Thunderstorm-derived lightning is a concern at higher elevations. Peaks, ridgetops, and tall trees may attract lightning strikes. It's best to get to lower elevations and avoid being the highest object in your area during thunderstorms.

Trail Essentials

- Spare cold-weather clothing
- Plenty of water
- Adequate food (plus a little more)

Less Than Essential, But Useful

Map and Compass (And the know-how to use them.) Many trails don't require much navigation, meaning a map and compass aren't always as essential as water or food—but it can be a close call. If the trail is remote or infrequently visited, a map and compass should be considered necessities. As the budgets of federal and state land management agencies have declined, so have the frequency and reliability of trail signs, as well as maintenance of the trails themselves.

A hand-held GPS is also a useful trail companion, but is really no substitute for a map and compass; knowing your longitude and latitude is not much help without a map.

Cell Phone Most parts of the country, even remote destinations, have some level of cellular coverage, particularly on peaks and ridgetops. In extreme circumstances, a cell phone can be a lifesaver. But don't depend on it; coverage is unpredictable and batteries fail.

Gear Depending on the remoteness and rigor of the trail, there are many additional useful items to consider: pocketknife, flashlight, fire source (water-proof matches, lighter, or flint), and a first-aid kit. Always carry some toilet paper and a light plastic trowel in case there is a need to go in the woods. Bury your waste at least 6 inches deep and more than 300 feet away from all water sources. Also, bring extra plastic bags to carry your used toilet paper out for proper disposal. A hiking staff or walking poles may enhance your experience by reducing the load on your feet and legs. Small binoculars are useful for viewing and identifying wildlife.

Every member of your party should carry the appropriate essential items described above; groups often split up or get separated along the trail. Solo hikers should be even more disciplined about preparation, and carry more gear. Traveling solo is inherently more risky. This isn't meant to discourage solo travel, simply to emphasize the need for extra preparation. Solo hikers should make a habit of carrying a little more gear than absolutely necessary.

Trail Etiquette

The overriding rule on the trail is "leave no trace." Interest in visiting natural areas continues to increase in North America, even as the quantity of unspoiled natural areas continues to shrink. These pressures make it ever more critical that we leave no trace.

Never Litter If you carried it in, it's easy enough to carry it out. Leave the trail in the same, if not better condition than you find it. Try picking up any litter you encounter and packing it out if possible.

Stay on the Trail Paths have been created, sometimes over many years, for many purposes: to protect the surrounding natural areas, to avoid dangers, and to provide the best route. Leaving the trail can cause damage that takes years to undo. Never cut switchbacks. Shortcutting rarely saves energy or time, and it takes a terrible toll on the land, trampling plant life and hastening erosion. Moreover, safety and consideration intersect on the trail. It's hard to get truly lost if you stay on the trail.

Share the Trail The best trails attract many visitors and you should be prepared to share the trail with others. Do your part to minimize impact.

Many of the trails in this book are used by hikers, mountain bikers, and equestrians. Some of the non-wilderness trails are even open to motorized use. Commonly accepted trail etiquette dictates that motor vehicles and bike riders yield to both hikers and equestrians, hikers yield to horseback riders, downhill hikers yield to uphill hikers, and everyone stays to the right. Not everyone knows these rules of the trail, so let common sense and good humor be the final guide.

Leave It There Destruction or removal of plants and animals, or historical, prehistoric or geological items, is certainly unethical and almost always illegal.

Follow Campfire Rules Many of the higher-elevation areas are off-limits to campfires due to high use and impacts on local vegetation from wood gathering. Lower-elevation areas may have seasonal campfire prohibitions during dry periods to reduce the chance of starting a wildfire. Check with the management agency before your outing for permanent and seasonal rules.

Trail Etiquette

- Leave no trace—never litter.
- Stay on the trail—never cut switchbacks.
- Share the trail—use courtesy and common sense.
- Leave it there—don't disturb wildlife.

Getting Lost If you become lost on the trail, stay on the trail. Stop and take stock of the situation. In many cases, a few minutes of calm reflection will yield a solution. Consider all the clues available; use the sun to identify directions if you don't have a compass. If you determine that you are indeed lost, remain on the main trail and stay put. You are more likely to encounter other people if you stay in one place.

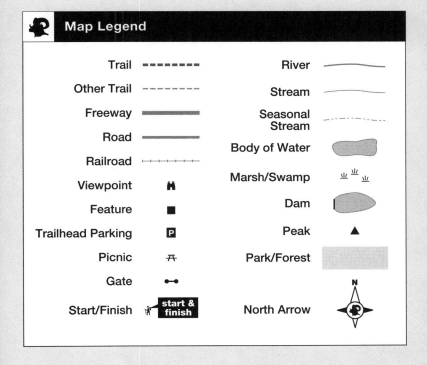

Map Legend

Trail	-------	River	
Other Trail	-------	Stream	
Freeway		Seasonal Stream	
Road		Body of Water	
Railroad			
Viewpoint		Marsh/Swamp	
Feature	■	Dam	
Trailhead Parking	P	Peak	▲
Picnic		Park/Forest	
Gate			
Start/Finish	start & finish	North Arrow	

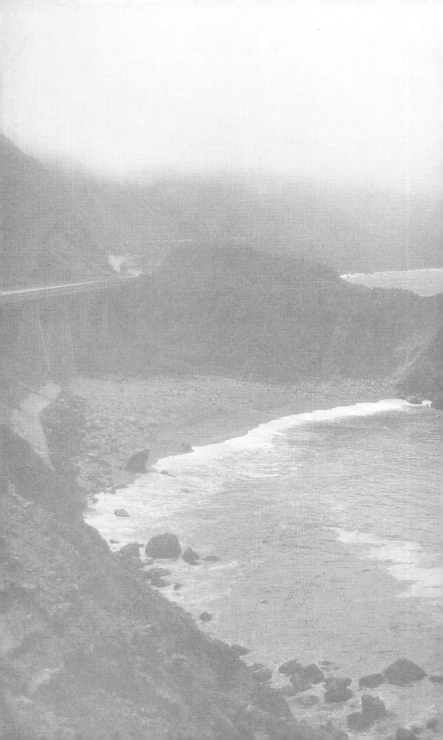

Southern Monterey County– Ragged Point

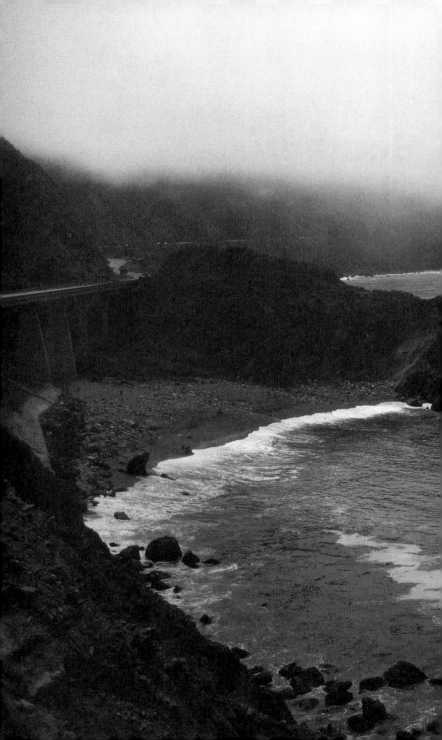

Southern Monterey County– Ragged Point

Ragged Point is small tourist stop tucked away in the northwest corner San Luis Obispo County, and few make the drive up Hwy. 1 to the Big Sur gateway unless they're traveling into Monterey County. From Ragged Point, the actual point is located a couple miles south of the small community of the same name, the rugged coast paralleling the highway north to southern Big Sur is as stunning as any in the Golden State.

Everyone knows just how beautiful the Big Sur area is. This chapter focuses on the often overlooked stretch that leads up to Big Sur, running from San Carpoforo Creek (also called San Carpojo Creek) at Ragged Point to majestic McWay Cove, where an 80-foot waterfall welcomes visitors to Julia Pfeiffer Burns State Park.

Hwy. 1 is a windy, two-lane road that gets clogged with campers and RVs in the summer. It can get washed out or covered by rockslides during the rainy season as well. Contact the Big Sur Ranger Station at (831) 667-2315 for current road conditions.

From San Carpoforo Creek, located 14 miles north of Hearst Castle, the highway carves into the Santa Lucia Mountain Range, which rises an average of 3,000 feet within 3 miles of the ocean. Some of the mountain peaks, including Cone Peak, top the 5,000-foot mark. As the highway climbs, the countless vista points and turnouts along the way offer gorgeous panoramas of the rocky cliffs that jut out into the Pacific. The seven trails in this chapter allow hikers get up close and personal with this dramatic stretch of coastline.

Overleaf and opposite: *Rockwell Landing at Limekiln State Park was once a shipping port.*

Permits and Maps

Most of the backcountry trails in Northern San Luis Obispo County and Southern Monterey County are located within the Los Padres National Forest. Trail maps and permit information can be picked up at the Big Sur Station. A National Forest Adventure Pass is required for some Los Padres hikes, although the program is being phased out in some areas. The pass can be purchased at ranger stations and area sporting goods retailers, including Big 5 in San Luis Obispo and Paso Robles. The $30 passes also can be ordered by calling (909) 382-2622.

Los Padres National Forest maps can be viewed at www.fs.fed.us/r5/for-estvisitormaps/lospadres or purchased at www.nationalforeststore.com. For more information, contact the Los Padres ranger station in Goleta at (805) 968-6640.

Day-use fees are charged at all of the main parks in the Big Sur area, including Julia Pfeiffer Burns (McWay Falls) and Limekiln (Limekiln Creek hikes) state parks. Save your day-use receipt, as it can be used to enter the other state parks in the area. Maps on specific hikes located within state parks can be picked up at the respective park's entrance kiosk.

There is no day-use fee for the hikes to Cone Peak, Jade Cove, Salmon Creek Falls, or San Carpoforo Creek.

The Ragged Point Nature Trail, which zigzags down to a cove located just north of Ragged Point Inn, is on hotel property, and the owner may restrict access at any time. The nature trail is free, although stopping by the snack bar for lunch or a coffee is a good way to keep the owner happy and keep the trail open to visitors.

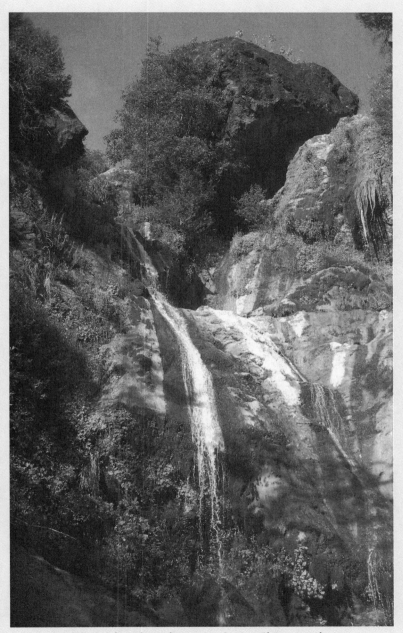

Salmon Creek Falls is located near the Monterey-San Luis Obispo county line.

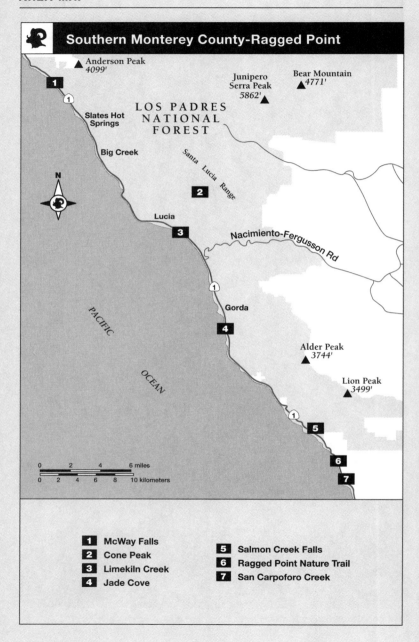

Southern Monterey County-Ragged Point

▲ Anderson Peak
4099'

1

①

Slates Hot
Springs

Junipero
Serra Peak
5862' ▲

Bear Mountain
▲*4771'*

LOS PADRES
NATIONAL
FOREST

Big Creek

Santa Lucia Range

2

Lucia

3

Nacimiento-Fergusson Rd

N

PACIFIC

①

Gorda

4

OCEAN

Alder Peak
▲ *3744'*

Lion Peak
▲*3499'*

①

5

6

7

| 0 | 2 | 4 | 6 miles |
| 0 | 2 | 4 | 6 | 8 | 10 kilometers |

1 McWay Falls

2 Cone Peak

3 Limekiln Creek

4 Jade Cove

5 Salmon Creek Falls

6 Ragged Point Nature Trail

7 San Carpoforo Creek

TRAIL FEATURE TABLE

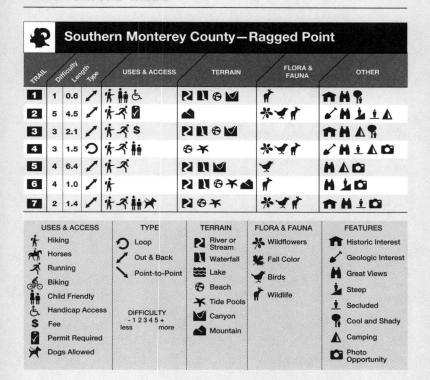

Southern Monterey County—Ragged Point

TRAIL	Difficulty	Length	Type	USES & ACCESS	TERRAIN	FLORA & FAUNA	OTHER
1	1	0.6	↗	🚶👫♿	🌊💧☀🏜	🦌	🏛🏔🌳
2	5	4.5	↗	🚶🏃✅	⛰	🌸🐦🦌	✏🏔💧🛑🏕
3	3	2.1	↗	🚶🏃$	🌊💧☀🏜		🏛🏔🏕🌳
4	3	1.5	↻	🚶🏃👫	☀✈	🌸🐦🦌	✏🔭💧🏕📷
5	4	6.4	↗	🚶🏃	🌊💧🏜	🐦	🔭🏕📷
6	4	1.0	↘	🚶	🌊💧☀✈⛰	🦌	🏔💧📷
7	2	1.4	↗	🚶🏃👫🐕	🌊☀✈	🌸🐦🦌	🏛🏔💧📷

USES & ACCESS	TYPE	TERRAIN	FLORA & FAUNA	FEATURES
🚶 Hiking	↻ Loop	🌊 River or Stream	🌸 Wildflowers	🏛 Historic Interest
🐎 Horses	↗ Out & Back	💧 Waterfall	🍁 Fall Color	✏ Geologic Interest
🏃 Running	↘ Point-to-Point	〰 Lake	🐦 Birds	🏔 Great Views
🚲 Biking		☀ Beach	🦌 Wildlife	🪜 Steep
👫 Child Friendly		✈ Tide Pools		🪧 Secluded
♿ Handicap Access	DIFFICULTY	🏜 Canyon		🌳 Cool and Shady
$ Fee	- 1 2 3 4 5 +	⛰ Mountain		🏕 Camping
✅ Permit Required	less more			📷 Photo Opportunity
🐕 Dogs Allowed				

Southern Monterey County–Ragged Point

The short but sweet McWay Falls Overlook Trail is ideal for people of all ages and hiking abilities. This trouble-free trail leads to a lookout from which you'll gaze across the cove to an 80-foot waterfall that is one of the most spectacular sights the Big Sur Coast has to offer.

The hike to Cone Peak is one of the most challenging climbs in southern Monterey County. The ridge rises immediately from the sea to an elevation of 5,155 feet, making up the steepest coastal elevation change in the continental United States.

This trail follows Limekiln Creek upstream to a trio of tributaries. The different legs of the hike end at an old redwood grove, and at Limekiln Falls and the historic lime kilns for which the state park is named.

This remote cove is popular with divers and jade collectors, but it is often overlooked by hikers because there is no trailhead kiosk or signed parking area. The free hike leads down to a rocky beach where the ragged coastline meets the turquoise surf.

Salmon Creek Falls................... 51

A spectacular, roadside waterfall is located within the first 0.25 mile of the trail, but few hikers realize they'll come to a second cascade, Upper Salmon Creek Falls, a couple miles upstream.

TRAIL 5

Hike, Run
6.4 miles, 3.0 hours
Out & Back
Difficulty: 1 2 3 **4** 5

Ragged Point Nature Trail 55

This nature trail, on the property of Ragged Point Inn, zigzags down a sketchy, 335-foot cliff to a remote cove below where otters play about in the kelp beds. Three-hundred-foot Black Swift Falls tumbles down the cliff face to the beach and can be seen in full view from there.

TRAIL 6

Hike
1.0 mile, 1.0 hour
Out & Back
Difficulty: 1 2 3 **4** 5

San Carpoforo Creek 61

This creekside trail follows San Carpoforo Creek as it spills out of the Santa Lucia Mountains and dumps into the ocean near Ragged Point. The second half of the trail is a beach hike along one of the few accessible sand beaches in southern Monterey County.

TRAIL 7

Hike, Run
1.4 miles, 1.0 hour
Out & Back
Difficulty: 1 **2** 3 4 5

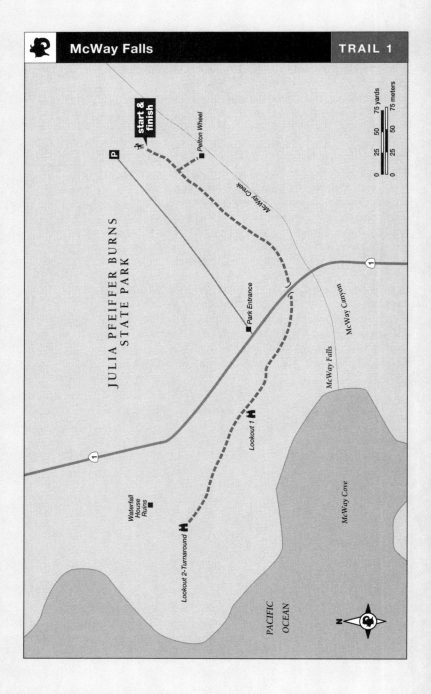

McWay Falls   TRAIL 1

start & finish

P

Pelton Wheel

McWay Creek

1

Park Entrance

McWay Canyon

JULIA PFEIFFER BURNS
STATE PARK

McWay Falls

Lookout 1

1

Waterfall
House
Ruins

Lookout 2-Turnaround

McWay Cove

PACIFIC
OCEAN

N

0   25   50   75 yards
0   25   50   75 meters

McWay Falls

One of Big Sur's most spectacular sights, McWay Cove at Julia Pfeiffer Burns State Park also is one of the region's most accessible destinations. The popular McWay Falls Overlook Trail is a relatively flat, trouble-free hike that spans less than 0.3 mile and ends with the best view of McWay's centerpiece—an 80-foot waterfall that pirouettes down a granite precipice to the white sandy beach below.

Best Time

The waterfall is most impressive after the rains die down. Water clarity improves in the spring and early summer, before school lets out and vacationers bombard the trail. The best time to spot migrating whales from the overlook is early in the year, although inclement weather and landslides can shut down Hwy. 1 during the winter months.

Finding the Trail

The day-use park is nestled along the Big Sur Coast about 37 miles south of Carmel and 55 miles north of San Simeon on Hwy. 1. The entrance to Julia Pfeiffer Burns State Park—not to be confused with the main campground located to the north at Pfeiffer Big Sur State Park—is clearly marked on the east side of the highway. The trailhead is near the entrance of the small parking area and originates alongside McWay Creek, a main waterway that passes through the heart of the park.

TRAIL USE
Hike

LENGTH
0.6 mile, 0.5 hour

VERTICAL FEET
±50 feet

DIFFICULTY
– **1** 2 3 4 5 +

TRAIL TYPE
Out & Back

SURFACE TYPE
Dirt

FEATURES
Handicap Access
Child Friendly
Canyon
Beach
Stream
Waterfall
Wildlife
Historic
Great Views
Cool & Shady

FACILITIES
Restrooms
Picnic Tables

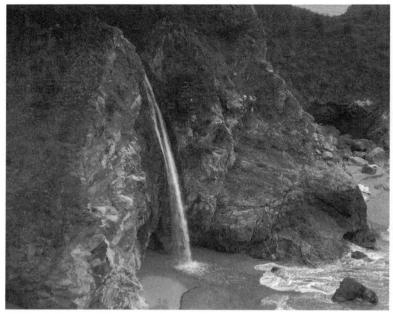

McWay Falls *is one of the most popular stops along the Big Sur coast.*

Trail Description

McWay Canyon is named after Christopher McWay, who made this his homestead here in the late 1870s before selling his Saddle Rock Ranch to former New York congressman Lathrop Brown in the 1920s.

Near the entrance to the day-use parking lot, find the sign marked WATERFALL OVERLOOK TRAIL ▶1 and head down the dirt path that parallels McWay Creek. At the onset of the hike is a turnoff to the Pelton Wheel, which is only 50 feet off the main path and worth a quick visit on the hike back. Continue straight on the main trail to a tunnel ▶2 that runs under Hwy. 1 at .08 mile. Stay right as you come out of the tunnel, and the first glimpse of the majestic cascade is to the left at .17 mile.

This main stem of the trail overlooks redwood, tan oak, and madrone chaparral, ending at the viewpoint ▶3 at 0.3 mile. There is a bench at 0.2 mile and two more benches at the turnaround, all of which make nice picnic stops.

While slender **McWay Falls** is the main draw, the rest of the cove is equally jaw dropping, with its smooth sand spilling into a turquoise surf zone that looks as if it's been lifted from a Hawaiian postcard. With otters frolicking about the kelp strands below, and an outside chance you'll witness gray whales, it's easy to see why most visitors to McWay Cove miss the last remaining remnants of the **Waterfall House**. The ruins of the house, owned by Lathrop and Helen Hooper Brown in the 1940s, are near the end of the trail. This area was a popular getaway for a good friend of the Browns, Big Sur pioneer Julia Pfeiffer Burns.

When you're done taking in all the cove has to offer, retrace your steps ▶4 to the beginning of the trail where you can check out the Pelton Wheel, which helped provide electricity for the nearby Saddle Rock Ranch in the 1930s.

Gray whales can be seen passing through the Big Sur area from December through April. From December to early February, gray whales can often be seen migrating to the south; in late February, they begin migrating back to Alaska with their newborns at their sides. They often seek refuge near the coastline and coves to protect their young from great white sharks and orca whales.

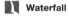 **Waterfall**

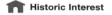 **Historic Interest**

🚶	**MILESTONES**	
▶1	0.0	Start at trailhead and proceed straight past the turnoff to Pelton Wheel.
▶2	0.1	Head through the tunnel and stay right, with the cove to your left.
▶3	0.3	The overlook marks the trail's end.
▶4	0.4	Return way you came, briefly stopping at the Pelton Wheel.

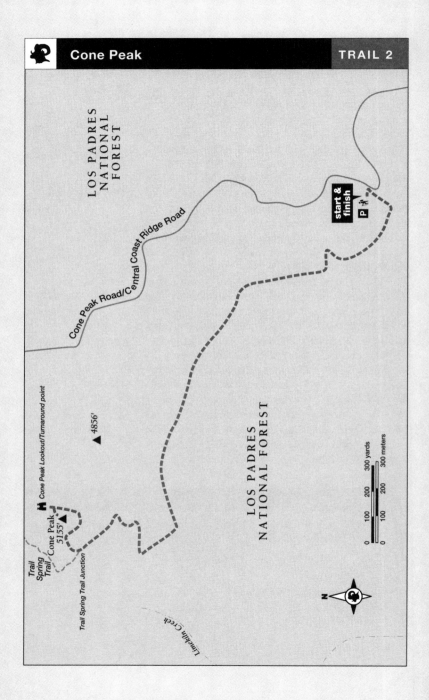

LOS PADRES
NATIONAL
FOREST

Cone Peak Road/Central Coast Ridge Road

start &
finish

LOS PADRES
NATIONAL FOREST

Cone Peak Lookout/Turnaround point

▲ 4856'

Trail
Spring
Trail

Cone Peak
5155' ▲

Trail Spring Trail Junction

Limekiln Creek

N

0   100   200   300 yards
0   100   200   300 meters

Cone Peak

This area is what Portuguese explorer Juan Rodríguez Cabrillo must have referred to in 1542 when he wrote that the Big Sur coast is made up of "mountains that seem to reach the heavens and the sea beats on them."

Cone Peak certainly fits the description, rising as it does from the sea to an elevation of 5,155 feet—making up one of the steepest coastal elevation changes in the United States. In fact, Cone Peak, which offers 360-degree views of the Ventana Wilderness, is the highest Los Padres National Forest summit next to nearby Junipero Serra (5,962 feet) and Pinyon (5,264 feet) peaks.

While the hike to Cone Peak isn't as grueling as the 12-mile trek to Junipero Serra, it is one of the most challenging hikes in Monterey County, as even the drive to the trailhead alone is tiring. But the solitude and peacefulness found on this remote hike are worth a couple of blisters and a dust-caked windshield.

Best Time

The dirt fire road to Cone Peak is often closed to vehicles during the rainy season, which generally leaves the trailhead open from May through November. The hike to Cone Peak is a typical inland peak trail, which is dry and in full sun for a majority of the hike.

TRAIL USE
Hike, Run

LENGTH
4.5 miles, 2.5 hours

VERTICAL FEET
±1405

DIFFICULTY
– 1 2 3 4 **5** +

TRAIL TYPE
Out & Back

SURFACE TYPE
Dirt

FEATURES
Permit Required
Mountain
Steep
Birds
Wildflowers
Wildlife
Great Views
Camping
Secluded
Geologic

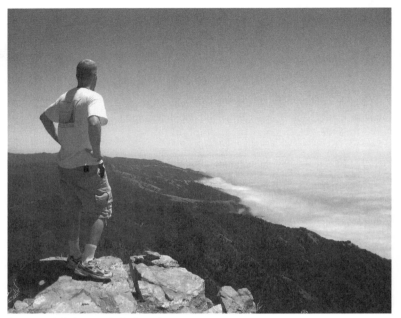

Cone Peak *lookout sits high above the Big Sur coast.*

Finding the Trail

From the Kirk Creek Campground along Hwy. 1—about 36 miles north of San Simeon—take Nacimiento–Fergusson Road for 7.0 miles to Cone Peak Road. Take the single-lane dirt road, also called Central Coast Ridge Road, for 5.0 miles to the turnout at the signed Cone Peak trailhead. The fire road is actually 6.0 miles long, so if you reach a dead end, you've driven past the trailhead.

Trail Description

The ascent to the peak is pretty straightforward, with signs at each of the junctions to help you avoid taking the wrong path. The lookout atop **the summit** gives hikers a visual to follow for much of the

 Steep

hike, which starts off at 3,716 feet ▶1 and parallels the fire road before coming to a saddle at 0.15 mile that overlooks the breathtaking Big Sur coastline. And this is just the start of the stellar viewpoints.

The trail offers the first inland views at 0.35 mile, looking out over the San Antonio and Nacimiento valleys. The reservoir to the southeast is Lake San Antonio. The trail hits the 4,000-foot mark at 0.45 mile, where you can look up at the old fire lookout at the summit.

Hike with caution over the next couple of miles, as eroding granite covers portions of the trail with dicey gravel. ▶2

At 1.2 miles, the trail passes through a manzanita grove that is still trying to bounce back from devastating fires that broke out during each of the previous three decades. The area was hit by the Marble Cone fire in 1978, the Rat Creek blaze in 1986, and the Kirk Complex fire in 1999. The fires have left many of the mature manzanita trees barren and ash-colored, although the native Santa Lucia firs and sugar pines at this elevation appear to be faring well.

The trail pulls away from the cliff's edge at 1.4 miles ▶3 and passes a towering sugar pine. The tree can be identified by its long, straight branches that are weighed down on the end by elongated cones. This is where the path really climbs, following a series of switchbacks and gaining 620 feet over the final 0.85 mile.

At the 2.0-mile mark is a junction with the Trail Spring Trail. ▶4 Stay right, following the signed trail to Cone Peak Lookout, which you'll reach in another 0.25 mile.

At **the summit**, at 2.25 miles, ▶5 an old fire lookout provides stunning, expansive views of the coast, interior river valleys, and the Santa Lucia Mountain Range. This is the turnaround for the hike. Because these views might be the best the Big

An old fire lookout located atop Cone Peak offers expansive views of the Ventana Wilderness.

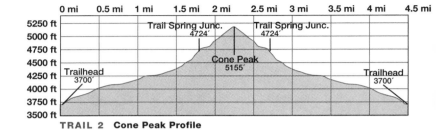

TRAIL 2 Cone Peak Profile

Sur coast has to offer, take your time before returning to the parking area via the same route.

Notice

An Adventure Pass, which can be picked up at sporting goods stores or ranger stations, is required for most Los Padres National Forest hikes.

There are no developed campgrounds or facilities within 12 miles of the trailhead. The closest facilities are at 33-site Kirk Creek Campground, at the Hwy. 1/Nacimiento–Fergusson Road junction, so bring plenty of water.

🚶 MILESTONES		
▶1	0.00	Start at trailhead next to parking area.
▶2	0.50	Hike with caution over gravelly stretch.
▶3	1.40	Trail veers away from cliff edge.
▶4	2.00	Stay right toward overlook at Trail Spring junction.
▶5	2.25	The peak marks the turnaround; return via same path.

Single-Track Trails

OPTIONS

If you have the energy for another hike, there are plenty of single tracks that are accessible via Cone Peak Road. A handful of trails and camps start at the trailhead at the end of 6.0-mile Cone Peak Road, including the popular Coast Ridge Trail. The Coast Ridge Trail follows a boulder-lined gully for 1.5 miles and offers nice views of the Big Sur coast along the way.

Starting off at the Coast Ridge Trail, you can follow hikes to Ojito, Trail Spring, and Gamboa and Cook Springs camps. If you're looking for more hiking on the way back to the junction with Nacimiento–Fergusson Road, the Vincente Flat and San Antonio trailheads are located at turnouts along Cone Peak Road.

The Vincente Flat trailhead is 3.7 miles from Nacimiento-Fergusson Road, on the west side of Cone Peak Road, and the San Antonio Trailhead is 4.0 miles from Nacimiento–Fergusson, on the east side of Cone Peak Road. The Vincent Flat Trail is a grueling point-to-point hike that starts at Cone Peak Road and descends nearly 8.0 miles to Hwy. 1, ending across the highway from the Kirk Creek Campground. Along the way, the trail descends more than 3,000 feet.

Just north of the Vincent Flat trailhead, the San Antonio Trail starts at Cone Peak Road and heads east to the headwaters of the Nacimiento and San Antonio rivers. The most popular stretch, to Fresno Camp, is 3.0 miles round-trip. Maps of this portion of the Los Padres National Forest can be purchased at Pacific Valley Station (30 miles north of San Simeon) along Hwy. 1. For more information, call (805) 927-4211.

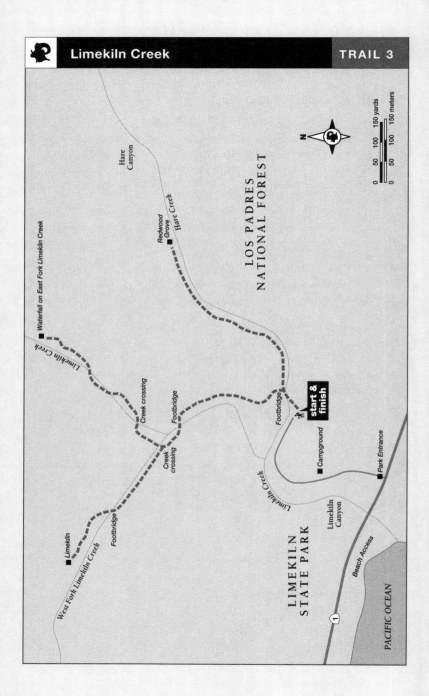

Limekiln Creek

TRAIL 3

Hare Canyon

Hare Creek

Redwood Grove

LOS PADRES NATIONAL FOREST

Waterfall on East Fork Limekiln Creek

Limekiln Creek

Creek crossing

Footbridge

Creek crossing

Footbridge

start & finish

Footbridge

Campground

Limekiln Creek

Park Entrance

Limekiln Canyon

Limekiln

West Fork Limekiln Creek

LIMEKILN STATE PARK

Beach Access

1

PACIFIC OCEAN

N

0   50   100   150 yards
0   50   100   150 meters

Limekiln Creek

This is really three 0.5-mile hikes rolled into one, following Limekiln Creek upstream to a trio of tributaries. The Hare Creek Trail follows its namesake to the northeast, traveling through Hare Canyon to a grove of mature redwoods. The other two trails wander to the northwest, one up to Limekiln Falls and the other to the historic limekilns that earned Limekiln State Park its name. Each path follows a shady redwood canyon and each holds an incentive at the end of a half-mile stroll.

Best Time

Because of the mild weather near the coast and the towering redwoods that provide shade throughout nearly the entire stretch of trails, there really isn't a bad time to hike at Limekiln State Park. Bring layered clothing when hiking near Big Sur. The park is open to day use from 8 a.m. to sunset. There are only a handful of parking spaces for day use, so the park recommends that hikers carpool when possible.

Finding the Trail

Limekiln State Park is near the small community of Lucia, on the east side of Hwy. 1, 56 miles south of Carmel and 94 miles north of San Luis Obispo. The parking area is near the restroom and campsite 23. Follow the creek upstream through campsites 23 through 34 to the trailhead, which is located at the north end of the park near the Limekiln Creek bridge. There is a day-use fee of $6.

TRAIL USE
Hike, Run
LENGTH
2.1 miles, 1.0 hour
VERTICAL FEET
±170
DIFFICULTY
– 1 2 **3** 4 5 +
TRAIL TYPE
Out & Back
SURFACE TYPE
Dirt

FEATURES
Parking Fee
Canyon
Stream
Waterfall
Beach
Cool & Shady
Great Views
Camping
Historic

FACILITIES
Restrooms
Water
Phone
Campground

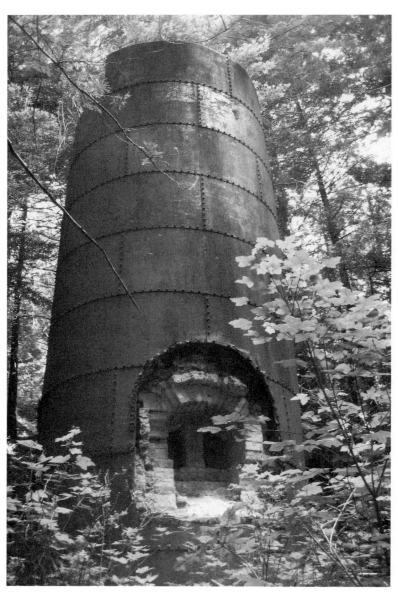

One of the old limekilns *for which the park is named*

Trail Description

Cross the bridge over Limekiln Creek to the initial fork in the trail. The right fork heads northeast up Hare Canyon to the Hare Creek Redwood Grove. The left fork travels northwest to the waterfall and limekilns.

Head right, following **Hare Creek** upstream ▶1 to the Sears and Roberts Grove, where a line of relatively young redwoods stands. While there are many redwoods that line these trails, the trees here are still relatively young after rebounding from heavy logging along the creek in the late 1800s. The trail ascends some rock steps at 0.2 mile, passing bright green ferns, thorny blackberry bushes, and moss-covered canyon walls.

You'll see a grove of mature redwoods at 0.3 mile, where the spur dead-ends ▶2 at a downed redwood and an END OF TRAIL sign. Head back to the initial fork in the trail. Reach the fork at 0.6 mile ▶3 and follow the path that follows Limekiln Creek upstream past the June and Pollack Grove. The trail runs into another fork after a footbridge crosses the creek at 0.85 mile.

Take the right spur, near the signed Harris Grove, to the East Fork. ▶4 The trail crosses the creek three times before reaching **Limekiln Falls** at 1.1 miles. ▶5 The majestic waterfall tumbles some 100 feet down the mossy limestone cliff. After soaking in the waterfall, return to the junction with the Limekiln Trail near the main creek, at 1.35 miles. ▶6

Head northwest up the final leg of the trail, which follows the West Fork up to the kilns for which the park is named at 1.6 miles. ▶7 This is where hikers can find the **remains of four stone and steel furnaces**, towering above the ferns and blackberry bushes that blanket the forest floor. Back in the 1800s, the base of a natural limestone deposit was transformed into a lime-manufacturing site for the Rockland Lime and Lumber Company, which

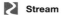 **Stream**

Look for the remains of four historic limekilns on the upper stretches of the West Fork of Limekiln Creek.

 Waterfall

Historic Interest

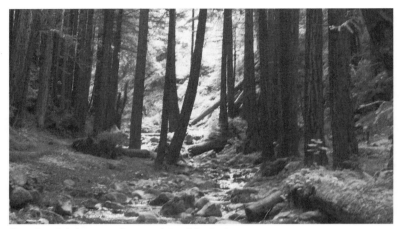

Hare Creek *before its confluence with Limekiln Creek*

fueled the furnaces with the seemingly endless sup-
ply of redwood in the area. The kilns helped "slake"
or purify the limestone, which was then shipped
by wagon down to the beach at Rockland Landing.
The lime was then shipped up the coast to be used
commercially.

The limekilns mark the final turnaround spot.
Follow the trail, which traces the same wagon route
used by the Rockland Lime and Lumber Company,
back to the trailhead at 2.1 miles.

🚶	MILESTONES	
▶1	0.00	Cross footbridge and head up right fork to Hare Canyon.
▶2	0.30	Trail dead-ends at grove; head back to trailhead.
▶3	0.60	Near the trailhead, take the Limekiln Falls Trail junction.
▶4	0.85	At the fork, stay right on the spur toward waterfall.
▶5	1.10	Reach waterfall; return back to the main creek.
▶6	1.35	Take the Limekiln Trail.
▶7	1.60	Trail reaches the turnaround spot at the limekiln.

Notice

Hikers are warned not to hike off trail, as the canyon walls are slick and steep and the limekiln remains are very unstable. Poison oak also is common in the area.

Limekiln State Park

OPTIONS

Limekiln State Park isn't just a hikers paradise. The historic park, which sees fewer visitors than the larger Big Sur campgrounds, also is a quiet little campground with 33 developed sites—many of them along Limekiln Creek or tucked behind towering redwoods. The sites are small, but each has a picnic table, fire ring, and room for two vehicles. No RVs longer than 24 feet are permitted.

Campers and day users also can take advantage of the park's beach access, which is rare along this rugged stretch of coast. To reach the beach, park in the day-use area and hike south beneath the Hwy. 1 bridge to the mouth of Limekiln Creek. The beach is better known as Rockland Landing, and is where the barrels of purified limestone were once loaded onto boats and shipped up the coast to be used in cement and other commercial products. There is a day-use fee of $6. Call (800) 444-7275 for additional camping information.

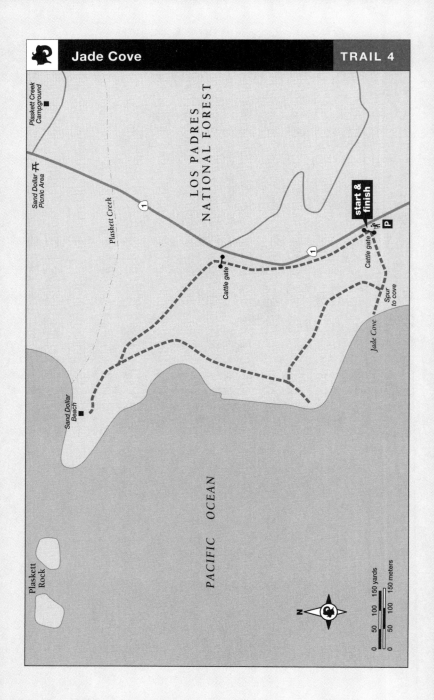

Jade Cove

TRAIL 4

LOS PADRES
NATIONAL FOREST

Plaskett Creek
Campground

Sand Dollar
Picnic Area

Plaskett Creek

1

start &
finish

P

Cattle gate

Cattle gate

Spur
to cove

Jade Cove

Sand Dollar
Beach

PACIFIC OCEAN

Plaskett
Rock

N

0   50   100   150 yards
0   50   100   150 meters

Jade Cove

This remote cove is where the gem that is Big Sur originates, but few know how to get here, as there is no trailhead kiosk or even a signed parking area. Hikers who find their way to the rocky beach are welcomed by rugged shore cliffs overlooking the turquoise surf between Cape San Martin to the south and Plaskett Rock to the north. The area is popular for divers hoping to find chunks of jade that have been polished by the pounding surf. But if diving isn't your thing, a spur down to the beach gives hikers a closer look at the rocky cove whose gravelly ocean floor is said to be sprinkled with bits of the greenish-colored nephrite.

Best Time

The trail is open all year, as long as two-lane Hwy. 1 is open up to Plaskett Creek Campground. The spur down to the cove gets slippery during the wet season, although it is still passable if hikers descend carefully. A negative tide is the best time to search the tide pools at the cove.

Finding the Trail

The Jade Cove access point is just south of Plaskett Creek Campground, about 15 miles north of Ragged Point and 30 miles north of San Simeon. The unsigned trailhead, essentially a cattle guard with steps that descend to a single track, is on the west side of Hwy. 1, directly across from the Jade Cove forest sign on the other side of the highway. Park in the turnout across from the sign.

TRAIL USE
Hike, Run
LENGTH
1.5 miles, 1.0 hour
VERTICAL FEET
±150
DIFFICULTY
– 1 2 **3** 4 5 +
TRAIL TYPE
Loop
SURFACE TYPE
Dirt

FEATURES
Child Friendly
Beach
Birds
Tide Pools
Wildflowers
Wildlife
Great Views
Photo Opportunity
Camping
Secluded
Geologic

45

Trail Description

 Beach

Step down the cattle guard and follow the single track toward the **beach**, making the loop in a clockwise direction. ►1 While there are no signs describing the trail or marking the trailhead, a sign near the start of the hike reminds hikers that prospecting, mining, or removal of any rock, mineral, or material is prohibited above mean high-tide level. Another sign warns of "life-threatening waves and currents," which keeps most divers and swimmers away.

Tide Pools

Within 500 feet of the trailhead, you reach the cliffs that overlook the rugged shore. From here, a steep spur descends to the rocky beach, which can be reached in 0.2 mile. After **exploring the cove**, climb back to the main path and follow the loop north toward Plaskett Creek. ►2

Follow the relatively flat track past the fragrant shrubs, coyote brush, and an interesting rock cluster on the east side of the trail. One triangular-shaped outcropping stands 15 feet above the meadow, ►3 looking like a gnomon (an indicator pin) on the face of a giant sundial. At the half-mile mark, the trail reaches another spur, with this one jutting out

Searching for Jade

NOTES

Jade in this area varies from black to green in color and is difficult to identify because it has many of the same characteristics as serpentine. Jade, however, is much harder and does not scratch easily.

Hikers should note that the U.S. Forest Service prohibits collecting jade above the mean high-tide line. That makes finding jade at this very rocky beach difficult for non-divers. The best bet for novice gem collectors is to shop for jade at the local shops in Big Sur. The Big Sur Jade Company has been collecting and selling jade since 1979, and jewelry makers put their work on display every fall at the Big Sur Jade Festival.

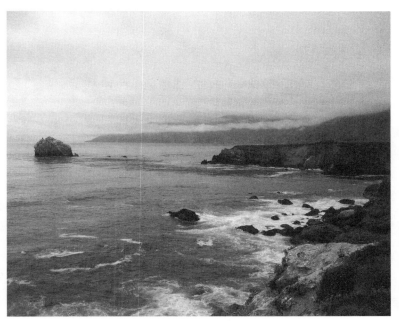

Dramatic Jade Cove, *just south of Plaskett Rock and campground*

to a point that offers remarkable views of Cape San Martin to the south and Plaskett Rock to the north. ▶4

Return to the main trail and continue north toward Plaskett Rock. Another jade-laden cove can be seen at the base of the cliffs at 0.75 mile. At 0.9 mile, the trail reaches the rocky finger pointing out to Plaskett Rock, ▶5 about 100 feet offshore. The guano-topped rock is another popular spot for divers searching for jade.

Plaskett Creek dumps into the Pacific just north of the rock. The creek helps bring nutrients to the inland vegetation, and its presence means the latter portions of the trail are often overgrown with thorny blackberry bushes and poison oak. If the trail has been cleared recently, it's possible to meander all

When conditions are calm, divers can find jade located off the shores of Jade Cove.

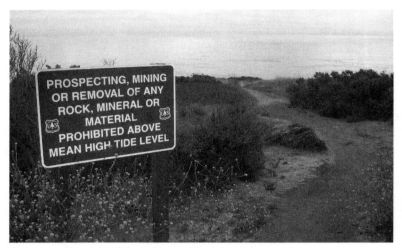

A sign near the start of the trail *warns hikers about jade removal.*

the way up to Sand Dollar Beach, although the safest bet is to continue following the trail back to the main highway.

The trail spits out at Hwy. 1 at the 1.2-mile mark. ►6 From here, hikers can go back the way they came and return to the car at 2.4 miles, or finish out the loop by following the highway south for 0.3 mile to the parking area. Hwy. 1 is a busy, narrow road, so stick to walking along the dirt turnout/parking area during the final leg of the trip.

🚶	MILESTONES	
►1	0.0	Start at the cattle guard, following single track clockwise.
►2	0.2	Jade Cove can be reached via a spur at the cliff's edge.
►3	0.4	Path weaves through field, passing rock outcroppings.
►4	0.5	A spur leads to another point off the main trail.
►5	0.9	Trail reaches point that shoots out toward Plaskett Rock.
►6	1.2	Loop continues to a cattle guard to the north; follow highway south for 0.3 mile to parking area.

Plaskett Creek Campground

While there are no facilities available along the trail, Plaskett Creek Campground is less than a mile to the north. Plaskett Creek offers 45 campsites nestled among the large Monterey pines that line the tiny creek. Family campsites are filled on a first-come basis; group sites may be reserved ahead of time. The campground also has a handful of bicycle and hike-in sites.

Sand Dollar Beach, a popular surf spot and one of the few sandy stretches along the Big Sur Coast, is accessible via the opposite side of Hwy. 1. The park is run by the Los Padres National Forest's Monterey Ranger District. Contact the Parks Management Company at (805) 434-1996 for more information.

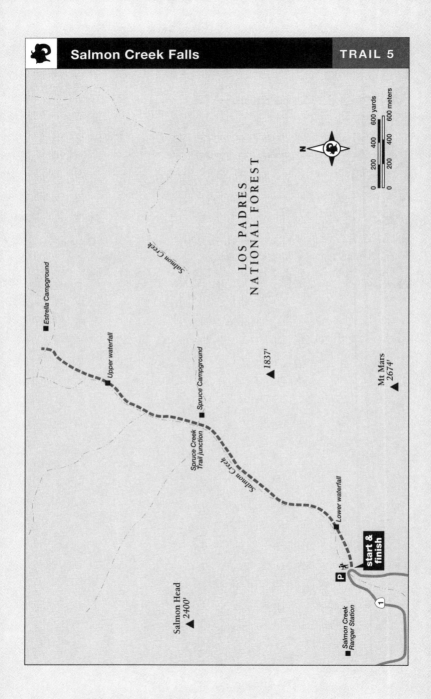

Estrella Campground

Upper waterfall

Salmon Creek

LOS PADRES
NATIONAL FOREST

N

0   200   400   600 meters
0   200   400   600 yards

Spruce Creek
Trail Junction

Spruce Campground

Salmon Creek

▲ 1837'

Mt Mars
▲ 2674'

Lower waterfall

start &
finish

P

Salmon Head
▲ 2400'

Salmon Creek
Ranger Station

1

Salmon Creek Falls

No trip to Big Sur would be complete without a stop at Salmon Creek Falls. The stunning, year-round waterfall is visible from Hwy. 1, so every third or fourth car usually stops for a quick peek. Few people make the short 0.2-mile hike to the base of the falls and even fewer make the 5.0-mile round-trip to Upper Salmon Creek Falls. But those who do get to experience two of the Central Coast's finest waterfalls on a single hike.

Best Time

Like many streams that are accessible by creekside trails, Salmon Creek is at its highest flows in the spring and early summer months. Salmon Creek gets bombarded with visitors during the vacation season, so morning hikes during the week are best for those hoping to avoid the crowds.

Finding the Trail

From Morro Bay, drive north on Hwy. 1 for 48 miles to the Monterey County line. The Salmon Creek Falls trailhead is located at the tight bend in the highway about 1.5 miles north of the San Luis Obispo County line and 8 miles south of Gorda. Park at the turnout on the east side of Hwy. 1, just before the old Forest Service station.

Trail Description

The most popular stretch of the hike runs from the highway to base of the lower falls, ▶1 which

TRAIL USE
Hike, Run
LENGTH
6.4 miles, 3.0 hours
VERTICAL FEET
±1110
DIFFICULTY
– 1 2 3 **4 5** +
TRAIL TYPE
Out & Back
SURFACE TYPE
Dirt

FEATURES
Canyon
Stream
Waterfall
Birds
Great Views
Photo Opportunity
Camping

FACILITIES
Picnic Tables

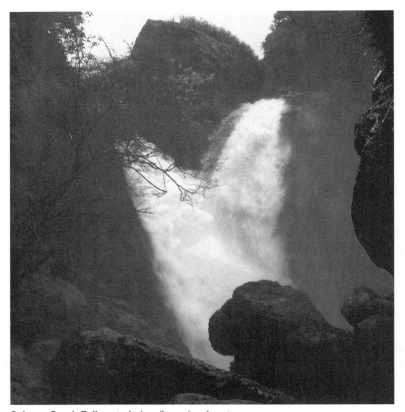

Salmon Creek Falls *at its highest flows after the rainy season*

is located at 0.1 mile. Start at the trailhead on the southern side of the creek and follow the clear-cut single track to the creek's edge and the base of the powerful 100-foot **waterfall**. After getting misted by the lower falls, retrace the trail to a junction with the single-track trail to Spruce Creek/Estrella Camp. ►2 The trail climbs more than 500 feet by the 0.3-mile mark and continues up to the flats along the banks of Salmon Creek.

The hike continues across seasonal **feeder creeks** and groves of Douglas firs. At 1.8 miles, the

Waterfall

Stream

trail passes the junction to Spruce Creek Trail, ►3
which runs to Dutra Flat (2.5 miles), Turkey Springs
(4.0 miles), and San Carpoforo (6.0 miles) camps.

Staying straight on the Salmon Creek Trail, the
path runs into Spruce Creek Camp ►4 at just over
2.0 miles.

Continue along the trail to forgotten-about
Upper Salmon Creek Falls. ►5 The waterfall is at
2.6 miles and, at 1,140 feet, nearly 1,000 feet higher
that the lower falls. After exploring the upper falls,
continue down the trail for another 0.5 mile to
Estrella Camp, which makes a good turnaround for
this hike because the trail is extremely overgrown
beyond this hike-in campground, which is at the
3.2-mile point. ►6 A picnic table at the camp makes
an ideal resting point for a break or picnic. Instead
of flirting with poison oak, return the way you came
to the trailhead and catch another glimpse of the
two falls on the way back.

 Camping

Notice

Hike-in camping is allowed at Spruce Creek, Estrella,
Dutra Flat, Turkey Springs, and San Carpoforo
camps.

🚶	**MILESTONES**	
►1	0.0	Start at the trailhead south of the creek.
►2	0.1	Enjoy the lower falls before backtracking to the trail to the upper campgrounds.
►3	1.8	Pass the junction to the Spruce Creek Trail.
►4	2.0	Trail rolls past Spruce Creek Camp.
►5	2.6	Another, lesser-known waterfall is visible.
►6	3.2	Reach Estrella Camp; head back the way you came.

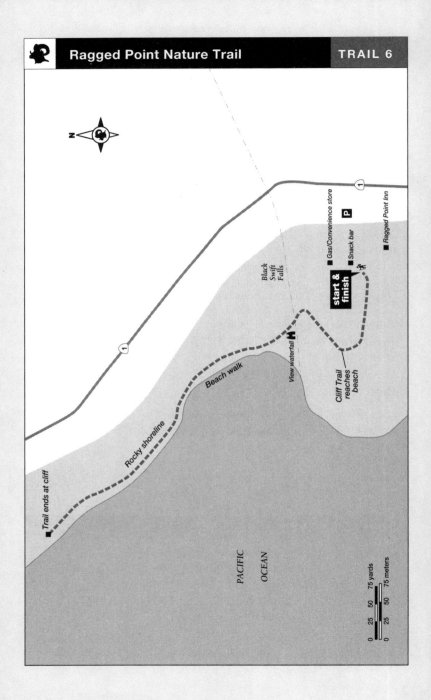

Ragged Point Nature Trail

TRAIL 6

1

Gas/Convenience store

P

Snack bar

Ragged Point Inn

Black
Swift
Falls

start &
finish

1

Cliff Trail
reaches
beach

View waterfall

Beach walk

Rocky shoreline

Trail ends at cliff

PACIFIC
OCEAN

0   25   50   75 yards

0   25   50   75 meters

Ragged Point Nature Trail

The Ragged Point Nature Trail is the northernmost trail among the San Luis Obispo County hikes. Its name is a bit deceiving in that the trail doesn't go to Ragged Point—the point is actually about 1.5 miles to the south, near the mouth of San Carpoforo Creek. Ragged Point, however, is the name of the community where the trail is located, a tourist stop known for its epic views of the rocky point to the south and the Big Sur coast to the north. The main draw here is Ragged Point Inn, a 30-room hotel that comes equipped with a restaurant, snack bar, mini-mart, and gas station.

Along with the amenities is a short but very steep nature trail that descends 335 feet to the beach. Via a handful of sketchy stairways and switchbacks, the narrow track zigzags down to black-sand beach that's reminiscent of the cove at San Carpoforo Creek.

While this tourist stop is popular with families, this trail is not for unsupervised children and should be hiked with extreme caution, as it's a long way down—evidenced by nearby Black Swift Falls, which tumbles more than 300 feet to the beach below.

TRAIL USE
Hike

LENGTH
1.0 mile, 1.0 hour

VERTICAL FEET
±330

DIFFICULTY
– 1 2 3 **4** 5 +

TRAIL TYPE
Out & Back

SURFACE TYPE
Dirt

FEATURES
Mountain
Steep
Stream
Waterfall
Beach
Tide Pools
Wildlife
Great Views
Photo Opportunity

FACILITIES
Restrooms
Picnic Tables
Water
Phone

Best Time

Because the creek doesn't always flow in the summer and fall, Black Swift Falls is most impressive in the spring. The trail, however, can be closed during wet weather. Avoid hiking on the trail around sunset, as it is tricky enough during daylight hours. The beach walk is made easier during a low tide.

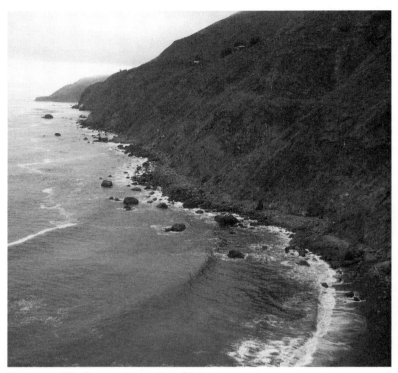

The rugged Big Sur coast, *near Ragged Point Inn*

Finding the Trail

The parking lot for Ragged Point Inn is on the west side of Hwy. 1, about 1.5 miles north of San Carpoforo Creek and 15 miles north of Hearst Castle. That's about 40 miles south of Big Sur, just a couple of miles past the San Luis Obispo County line. The signed trailhead is located near the gazebo in back of the restaurant.

Trail Description

From the outset, the trail descends a set of shaky wooden steps that will give hikers an idea of what to expect over the next quarter mile. ►1 The trail is short, but **drops 300 feet** in a hurry, so take your time on the way down.

 Steep

For those who don't believe they should make the entire hike, a bench is located near the base of the stairway. The bench offers grand views of the Big Sur coast to the north. An old handrail borders the trail after the bench, although trail users should rely on their own balance on this hike and not depend on any of the wooden steps or the structures that line the trail.

Ragged Point is visible protruding into the pounding surf about 1.5 miles south of the inn.

At 0.1 mile, the single track runs beneath a tree and stops at a saddle that makes for a nice vantage point. ►2 Follow the switchback and continue the descent to the black-sand cove below. The trail reaches a miniature grove of cypress trees at 0.2 mile. Then at the 0.25-mile mark, ►3 the trail spits out at the beach, where hikers can gaze back up and see just how far they've come. To the east, 300 feet above, is the start of **Black Swift Falls**. In the spring, the tiered waterfall pirouettes down the cliff face to the granite boulders below, where it eventually spills out into the Pacific Ocean.

 Waterfall

This trail can be extended to a full mile (round trip) with a short beach walk ►4 along with some rock hopping at the west end of the cove. The sandy **beach** runs into a rugged rock pile at the base of the cliff at 0.3 mile. The rusty remains of a car that once fell from the highway above can be seen at .35 mile. Continue boulder hopping to the turnaround spot at the 0.5-mile mark, ►5 where the surf runs right up against the cliff. Return the way you came.

 Beach

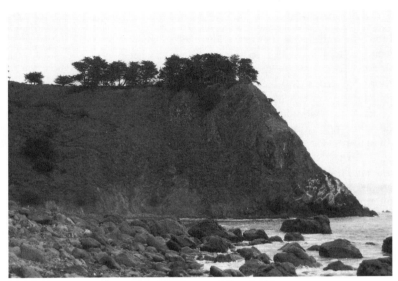

The nature trail carves its way *down the steep cliff north of the inn.*

Notice

The trail is located on hotel property, so the owner may restrict access at any time. The hike is not recommended for children, the elderly or novice hikers.

🚶	**MILESTONES**		
▶1	0.00	Descend the stairs.	
▶2	0.10	Trail passes beneath a tree.	
▶3	0.25	Trail reaches the beach.	
▶4	0.30	Continue west to end of the cove.	
▶5	0.50	Return the way you came.	

California Sea Otter

It's not rare to see a small raft of sea otters floating about the cove belly up, cracking open mussels, clams, and other invertebrates as they snack on their backs throughout the day.

California sea otters were once a common sight up and down the entire California coast and into Baja California until hunters nearly wiped them out by the late 1800s. By the early 1900s, until they stumbled upon a group of about 50 survivors in 1915, biologists feared the California subspecies—also known as the southern sea otter—had been hunted into extinction. Biologists kept this colony, which lived in a remote Big Sur cove, to themselves for more than 20 years, and the population began to bounce back. As of the summer of 2007, there were more than 3,000 otters on the Central Coast, all of which were believed to be descendants from that Big Sur colony.

While the sea otter population has grown, the numbers are nowhere near where they were before the fur trade, when more than 15,000 otters lived along the California coast. While California sea otters are protected as a threatened species under the 1972 Endangered Species Act, biologists suggest the southern species has been plagued of late by disease and by parasites stemming from coastal pollution. Biologists and local conservation groups fear continued pollution or a major oil spill in the area could wipe out the population completely now that the species is exclusive to the Central Coast.

Today, a majority of the sea otters can be found frolicking about the California Sea Otter Game Refuge, which runs from the Carmel River in Carmel to Santa Rosa Creek in Cambria.

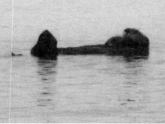

Sea otters often carry stones *to open shellfish on their bellies.*

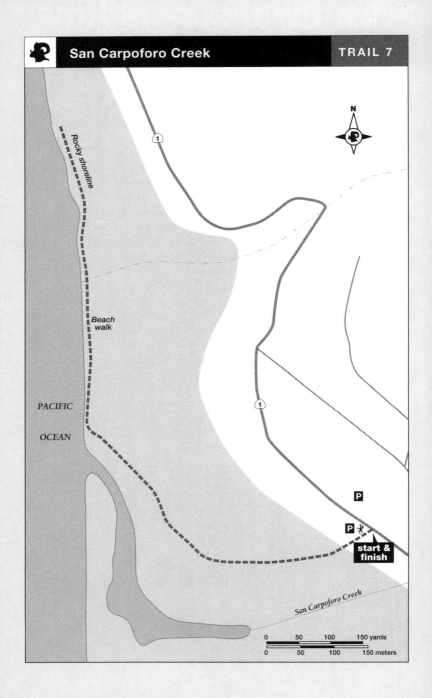

N

1

Rocky shoreline

Beach
walk

PACIFIC

OCEAN

1

P

P

start &
finish

San Carpoforo Creek

| 0 | 50 | 100 | 150 yards |
| 0 | 50 | 100 | 150 meters |

San Carpoforo Creek

This short but noteworthy creekside trail follows San Carpoforo Creek downstream to its confluence with the Pacific, where it flows along a spectacular stretch of shoreline that goes overlooked by many RVers hustling up Hwy. 1 to Big Sur.

Not that San Carpoforo goes completely unnoticed. In fact, the creek, just south of the community of Ragged Point, was the route of Gaspar de Portolá's 1769 expedition, which followed the creek on its way up to the Santa Lucia Mountains. This small but resource-filled freshwater wetland was an ideal camp, as its upper stretches provide spawning grounds for the southern steelhead.

Best Time

February is a fun time to visit this chunk of coastline, as it is mating season for the resident elephant seals, which can be found just south of the Piedras Blancas lighthouse. The temperatures are mild along the north coast of San Luis Obispo County, so the weather isn't much of a factor at this beach. Fog is usually the only climate-related obstacle along these parts. The beach walk portion of the trail is easier during a low tide.

Finding the Trail

From Morro Bay, head north on Hwy. 1 for about 40 miles. The creek is 4.0 miles north of the turnoff to Hearst Castle, about 2.0 miles south of the community of Ragged Point, near the Monterey County line. Follow the highway over the signed creek and

TRAIL USE
Hike, Run

LENGTH
1.4 miles, 1.0 hour

VERTICAL FEET
±45

DIFFICULTY
– 1 **2** 3 4 5 +

TRAIL TYPE
Out & Back

SURFACE TYPE
Dirt

FEATURES
Child Friendly
Dogs Allowed
Stream
Beach
Birds
Tide Pools
Wildflowers
Wildlife
Great Views
Photo Opportunity
Secluded
Historic

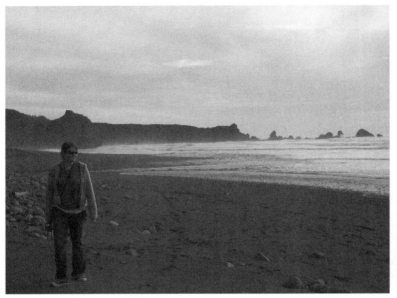

San Carpoforo Creek *meets the ocean just north of Ragged Point.*

park near the gate on the west side of the highway. The turnoff is located across the street from the ranch house. Do not block the gate and park well off the side of the busy highway. There are a pair of turnouts on the east side of the highway as well.

Trail Description

Pass alongside the gate and follow the well-defined but unsigned path down to the sandy beach. ▶1 Near the trailhead, you'll see a sign with information on the **western snowy plover**. Stay on the dirt single track for the first half of the trail, as the area between the trailhead and beach is a nesting area for the threatened bird.

The first 0.25 mile weaves through chaparral and creekside vegetation before giving way to the beach community. The exception to the waist-high

Birds

shrubbery is a massive cypress tree that towers above, 0.15 mile into the hike. A spur off to the left of the single track crawls beneath the cypress branches to a shaded den. From here you can escape the sun, bird-watch, and study the gnarled limbs branching off the mature tree. The crashing surf in the distance shows just how close the tree is to the beach and mouth of the creek.

Stay to the right of the **creek** and follow its flows to the beach, which can be reached in just under 0.5 mile. ▶2 This is where freshwater and saltwater worlds collide, in the topsy-turvy surf zone just north of the rocky finger nicknamed Ragged Point. From here, the trail is really a beach walk to the north. ▶3 If the tides allow, continue north to catch a preview of what the Big Sur coastline looks like.

Along the way, where water trickles down from the Santa Lucia Mountains, a couple of tiny coves offer a reprieve from the afternoon winds. At 0.55 mile, ▶4 an intermittent stream flows beneath a boulder-filled crevice to the ocean. The taller rocks provide good vantage points for the **marine life** in the area, which includes seals, otters, and dozens of seabirds.

The turnaround is located at 0.7 mile, ▶5 where massive boulders have tumbled down to the **beach** from the cliffs above. Head back the way you came, stopping to take in the sunset if you are on an evening hike. The beach near the mouth of San Carpoforo Creek is a perfect spot for sunsets, as from there it is only a short hike back to the car.

Notice

The creek also has been called San Carpojo Creek, and some old trail markers and maps still refer to it as such.

Along the beach portion of this hike, Ragged Point can be seen jutting out into the surf to the

San Carpoforo Creek leads to an accessible beach along the rugged coast.

 Stream

 Wildlife

 Beach

south. While the small community just north of San Carpoforo Creek also is named Ragged Point, the actual point is to the south.

Watch out for seals, which stack up in the surf zone in search of food. San Carpoforo Creek is a well-known steelhead passageway, and the San Simeon coastline is famous for its seals, including the enormous elephant seals that mate here early in the year. If you see a seal on the beach, give it space. Elephant seals are an aggressive (and protected) species.

MILESTONES

►1	0.00	Pass through the gate toward the beach.
►2	0.45	Trail runs alongside creek.
►3	0.50	Reach the mouth and follow the beach north.
►4	0.55	Cross over intermittent stream.
►5	0.70	Large boulders mark the turnaround.

Piedras Blancas Rookery

A popular rookery for the northern elephant seal can be found about 9.0 miles south of San Carpoforo Creek (5.0 miles north of the Hearst Castle turnoff). The turnoff to the day-use area and boardwalk walkway is on the west side of the highway; just look for all of the cars and signs.

The sandy beach rookery, just south of Piedras Blancas, is where more than 15,000 seals migrate for birthing, molting, and resting throughout the year. Visits from these enormous elephant seals peak three times annually—in January, after a majority of births have occurred; in April, during the peak molting period; and in October, during the juvenile haul-out.

The Piedras Blancas rookery is open to the public year-round during daylight hours. There are no admission fees or reservations required, and during the peak seasons, docents are on hand to teach visitors about the elephant seal.

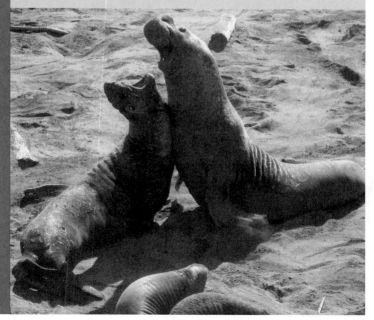

Elephant seals *are most active early in the year.*

CHAPTER 2

Northern San Luis Obispo County

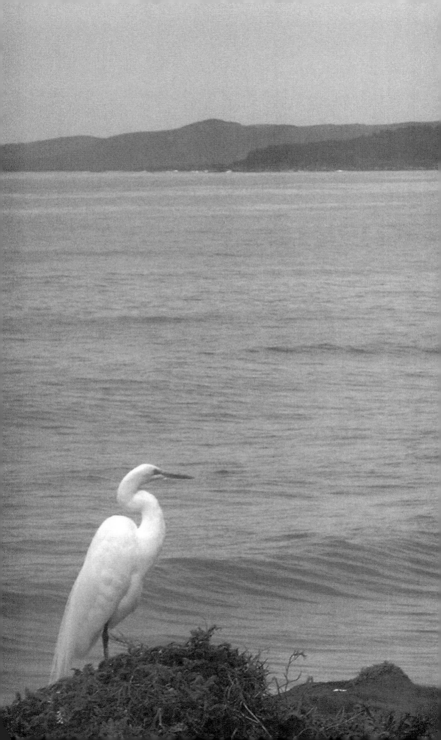

Northern San Luis Obispo County

San Luis Obispo County's north coast rivals Big Sur, offering some of the most pristine stretches of coastline in the Golden State. Why do you think William Randolph Hearst built his castle here? Speaking of Hearst, in 2004, California State Parks acquired 959 acres and 13 miles of coastline as part of the $95 million Hearst Ranch conservation deal. The agreement provides access to coastline that was previously off-limits to the public.

The San Simeon Point and Villa Creek trails give hikers a rare view of two north coast stretches that are void of housing developments and look very much the same as they did hundreds of years ago. South of Morro Rock, the most recognizable landmark on the Central Coast, hikers have all sorts of options at Morro Bay and Montaña de Oro state parks. The two parks bookend an estuary that is considered one of the top birding locations on the West Coast. Two ideal bird-watching spots are perched along the boardwalk hike into the 90-acre Elfin Forest, most of which was added to Morro Bay State Park in 1988. This boardwalk hike is one of the best wheelchair-accessible birding trails in the state.

For hikers looking for more of a challenge, the climbs to nearby Cerro Cabrillo and Cerro Alto provide expansive views of the county. When the fog blankets the coast, many hikers retreat inland, where the Jim Green Trail and Salinas River Parkway give North County residents much-needed trail access. Those looking for remote backcountry trails need to look no farther than the Santa Margarita Lake area, where the Rinconada and Blinn Ranch trails are open to hikers, mountain bikers, and equestrians. The 18-mile Blinn Ranch Trail is the longest trail in this guide, running along the perimeter of Santa Margarita Lake from the Salinas River near Pozo all the way to the dam area on the west side of the lake.

Overleaf and opposite: *A great white heron perched along the San Simeon coast.*

Permits and Maps

There is no day-use fee at William Randolph Hearst State Beach, where the trail to San Simeon Point begins. The kiosk at the beach is usually closed, so information on the beach is scarce. Try the Coastal Discovery Center near the pier, the Hearst Castle visitors center, or the San Simeon State Park entrance kiosk for more information. The public easement offering access to the point at San Simeon Cove was part of the Hearst Ranch conservation deal, and many of the trails included in the deal were still without signs and information kiosks when this guidebook went to press.

The trail to Villa Creek also was without a trailhead sign or information kiosk, although the bluff-top trail is free to the public and easy to navigate. A brochure on the hikes within Morro Bay State Park is available at the entrance kiosk to the campground, across from the marina. Montaña de Oro's many trails also are mapped on a brochure that's available at the visitors center near the campground. The Cerro Alto hikes are in the Los Padres National Forest at Cerro Alto Campground, which is under the direction of the Parks Management Company. A map of the many trails in the area is available at www.parksman.com.

A National Forest Adventure Pass is required for some Los Padres hikes, although the program is being phased out in some areas. The pass can be purchased at ranger stations and area sporting goods retailers, including Big 5 in San Luis Obispo and Paso Robles. The $30 passes also can be ordered by calling (909) 382-2622. Los Padres National Forest maps can be viewed at www.fs.fed.us/r5/forestvisitormaps/lospadres or purchased at www.nationalforeststore.com. For more information, contact the Los Padres ranger station in Goleta at (805) 968-6640.

The Jim Green (Atascadero) and Salinas River Parkway (Paso Robles) trails are maintained locally. Information is available through the respective city chamber of commerce or recreation department. The trails in this chapter that require a day-use fee are Cerro Alto and the Blinn Ranch Trail (trails 14 and 17). A comprehensive map of all the hikes in the Santa Margarita Lake area is available at the main entrance kiosk. A parking fee can be deposited at the kiosk near the parking area near the trailhead.

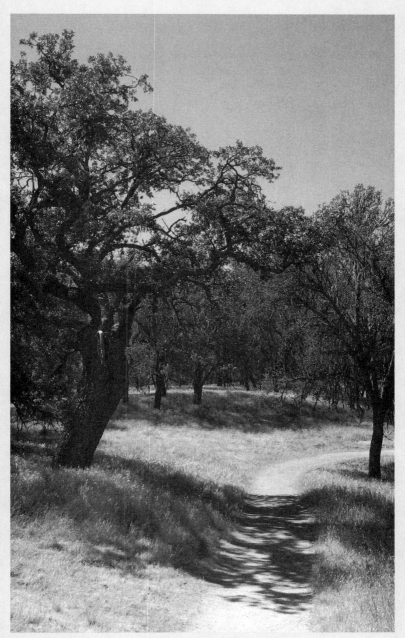

The Jim Green Trail *wanders beneath a canopy of oak trees.*

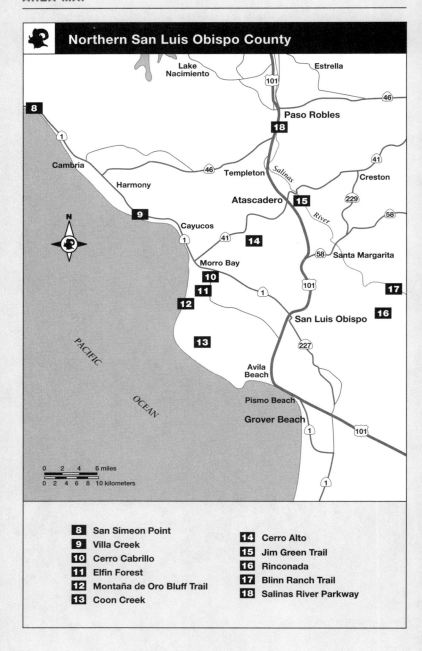

Northern San Luis Obispo County

8 San Simeon Point
9 Villa Creek
10 Cerro Cabrillo
11 Elfin Forest
12 Montaña de Oro Bluff Trail
13 Coon Creek

14 Cerro Alto
15 Jim Green Trail
16 Rinconada
17 Blinn Ranch Trail
18 Salinas River Parkway

TRAIL FEATURE TABLE

Northern San Luis Obispo County

TRAIL	Difficulty	Length	Type	USES & ACCESS	TERRAIN	FLORA & FAUNA	OTHER
8	3	2.5	Out & Back	Hiking, Running, Child Friendly	River or Stream, Beach, Tide Pools	Birds, Wildlife	Historic Interest, Steep, Secluded
9	2	2.4	Out & Back	Hiking, Running	Beach, Tide Pools	Wildflowers, Birds, Wildlife	Great Views, Steep, Photo Opportunity
10	4	2.5	Out & Back	Hiking, Horses, Running, Biking	Mountain	Wildflowers, Birds, Wildlife	Geologic Interest, Great Views, Steep, Secluded, Photo Opportunity
11	1	1.0	Loop	Hiking, Horses, Running, Biking, Child Friendly, Handicap Access, Dogs Allowed	Wetland	Birds, Wildlife	Great Views, Photo Opportunity
12	2	3.3	Out & Back	Hiking, Running, Biking, Child Friendly	Beach, Tide Pools	Wildflowers	Geologic Interest, Great Views, Steep
13	3	4.4	Out & Back	Hiking, Running	River or Stream	Wildflowers, Fall Color, Birds, Wildlife	Geologic Interest, Camping, Cool and Shady
14	4	4.0	Out & Back	Hiking, Horses, Running, Biking, Fee, Dogs Allowed	River or Stream, Canyon, Mountain	Birds	Great Views
15	2	1.7	Loop	Hiking, Horses, Running, Biking, Child Friendly, Dogs Allowed	Meadow	Wildflowers, Birds, Wildlife	Great Views
16	4	4.6	Loop	Hiking, Horses, Running, Biking, Dogs Allowed	River or Stream, Canyon, Mountain	Wildflowers, Birds, Wildlife	Historic Interest, Geologic Interest, Great Views, Photo Opportunity
17	5	18	Out & Back	Hiking, Horses, Running, Biking, Dogs Allowed, Permit Required	River or Stream, Lake	Wildflowers, Birds, Wildlife	Great Views, Steep, Camping
18	2	2.2	Out & Back	Hiking, Running, Biking, Child Friendly, Handicap Access, Dogs Allowed	River or Stream	Wildflowers, Fall Color, Birds, Wildlife	

Legend

USES & ACCESS
- Hiking
- Horses
- Running
- Biking
- Child Friendly
- Handicap Access
- $ Fee
- Permit Required
- Dogs Allowed

TYPE
- Loop
- Out & Back
- Point-to-Point

DIFFICULTY
- 1 2 3 4 5 +
- less — more

TERRAIN
- River or Stream
- Waterfall
- Lake
- Beach
- Tide Pools
- Canyon
- Mountain
- Wetland
- Meadow

FLORA & FAUNA
- Wildflowers
- Fall Color
- Birds
- Wildlife

FEATURES
- Historic Interest
- Geologic Interest
- Great Views
- Steep
- Secluded
- Cool and Shady
- Camping
- Photo Opportunity

Northern San Luis Obispo County

San Simeon Point 79
Starting off as a beach hike, the trail climbs the bluff to an old access road that leads to San Simeon Point, which offers unrivaled views of the cove, Hearst Castle, and San Simeon Pier.

Villa Creek 83
The unsigned bluff-top trail to Villa Creek travels through prime western snowy plover nesting habitat, running along the beach to the creek at Estero Bay.

Cerro Cabrillo 87
While Morro Rock and Hollister Peak are off-limits to the public, hikers and climbers can ascend 911-foot Cerro Cabrillo for awe-inspiring views of the estuary, coastline, and remaining chain of the Nine Sisters.

Elfin Forest. 93
One of the best wheelchair-accessible hikes in the area, this boardwalk trail loops around 90-acre Elfin Forest Natural Area, located on the south end of the estuary. Also, the trail offers some of the best views there are of Morro Bay.

Montaña de Oro Bluff Trail

The name of the trail says it all, as the dirt path runs along Montaña de Oro State Park's beachside bluffs, overlooking the pounding surf as it beats on the immaculate Diablo Canyon coast to the south. The constant battering of waves has carved spectacular rock outcroppings and even a few caves in the points that branch out into the surf.

TRAIL 12

Hike, Run, Bike
3.3 miles, 1.5 hours
Out & Back
Difficulty: 1 **2** 3 4 5

Coon Creek

Coon Creek tumbles along the southern perimeter of Montaña de Oro State Park before spilling into the Pacific just north of Point Buchon. It's believed the creek is named for the raccoons that inhabit the area, although you're more likely to see endangered steelhead from one of the many footbridges crossing the creek.

TRAIL 13

Hike, Run
4.4 miles, 2.0 hours
Out & Back
Difficulty: 1 2 **3** 4 5

Cerro Alto

Cerro Alto isn't one of the famed Nine Sisters, but you wouldn't know it by the view. On a clear day, views from the peak span all the way up the Estero Bay coast to Cambria and even San Simeon. This multiuse trail is one of only a few northern San Luis Obispo County trails open to mountain bikes, dogs, and horses.

TRAIL 14

Hike, Run, Bike, Horse
4.0 miles, 2.0 hours
Out & Back
Difficulty: 1 2 3 **4** 5

Jim Green Trail

A well-groomed county parks trail, the Jim Green Trail winds through moss-strewn oak trees and poppy-dotted hillsides before running alongside the lush greens of Chalk Mountain Golf Course in Atascadero.

TRAIL 15

Hike, Run, Bike, Horse
1.7 miles, 1.0 hour
Loop
Difficulty: 1 **2** 3 4 5

TRAIL 16

Hike, Run, Bike, Horse
4.6 miles, 2.5 hours
Loop
Difficulty: 1 2 3 **4** 5

Starting out near an abandoned mine, the Rinconada Trail climbs the Santa Margarita foothills of the Los Padres National Forest. It crosses flowery grasslands, chaparral shrublands, and oak woodlands before it descends to Little Falls Canyon and the headwaters of Little Falls Creek.

TRAIL 17

Hike, Run, Bike, Horse
18 miles, all day
Out & Back
Difficulty: 1 2 3 4 **5**

One of longest trails in San Luis Obispo County, Blinn Ranch Trail runs around the north side of Santa Margarita Lake, giving hikers, mountain bikers, and equestrians a glimpse of a side of the lake that is seldom explored by the public.

TRAIL 18

Hike, Run, Bike
2.2 miles, 1.0 hour
Out & Back
Difficulty: 1 **2** 3 4 5

Paso Robles needed a city trail like this, and a bond passed in 2002 helped bring plans for the Salinas River Parkway to fruition. The trail begins as a walk in the park before running beneath the Niblick Bridge and proceeding alongside the Salinas River.

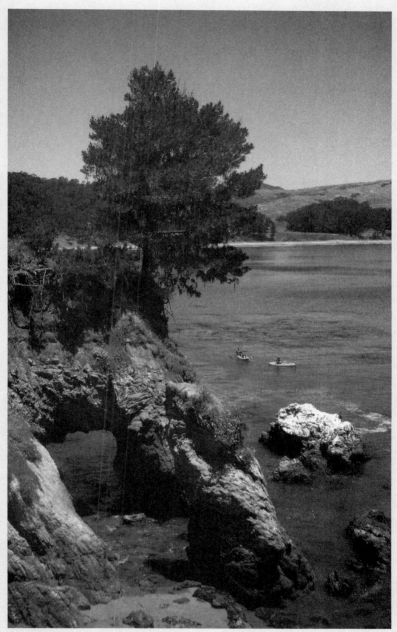

San Simeon Point *is a popular getaway for hikers and kayakers alike.*

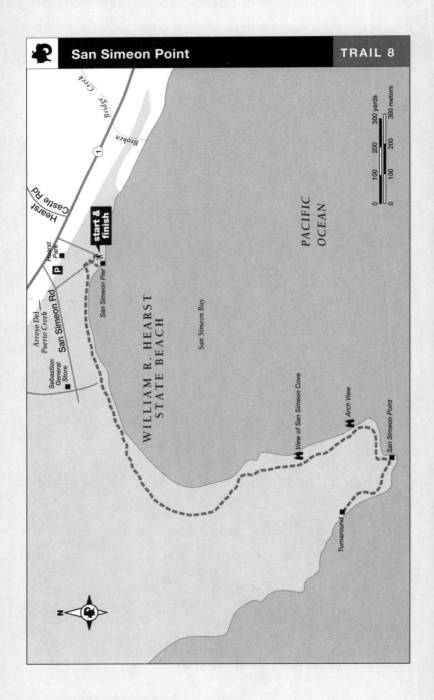

San Simeon Point

TRAIL 8

Bridge

Creek

Broken

1

Hearst Castle Rd

start & finish

Hearst Park

P

San Simeon Pier

Arroyo Del Puerto Creek

San Simeon Rd

Sebastian General Store

WILLIAM R. HEARST STATE BEACH

San Simeon Bay

PACIFIC OCEAN

View of San Simeon Cove

Arch View

San Simeon Point

Turnaround

N

0   100   200   300 yards
0   100   200   300 meters

San Simeon Point

This trail runs along the perimeter of the Hearst family's famous wharf, where tallow, hides, grain, and quicksilver were once exported from the ranch property. Today, William R. Hearst Memorial State Beach is an 8-acre park with a pier, picnic tables, and a popular beach. The trail begins as a beach walk but continues along a crescent of eucalyptus, pine, and cypress to San Simeon Point. Public access to the point is now permitted as part of a $95 million Hearst Ranch conservation deal.

Best Time

Because of the cool temperatures, there really isn't a bad time to hike here. The latter half of the trail is shaded by groves of oak, eucalyptus, and pine, providing a cool stretch of trail perfect for the dog days of summer.

Finding the Trail

Hearst Memorial State Beach is on the west side of Hwy. 1 about 8 miles north of Cambria, across the highway from the turnoff to Hearst Castle. Follow San Simeon Road for less than 0.25 mile to the park entrance. The large parking area (no fee) is on the left-hand side, near restrooms, a grassy picnic area, a nature center, and the beginning of the pier.

Trail Description

There isn't a distinct trailhead for this trail, but the pier is a good starting point. ▶1 Head north from

TRAIL USE
Hike, Run

LENGTH
2.5 miles, 1.5 hours

VERTICAL FEET
±70

DIFFICULTY
– 1 2 **3** 4 5 +

TRAIL TYPE
Out & Back

SURFACE TYPE
Dirt

FEATURES
Child Friendly
Stream
Beach
Birds
Tide Pools
Wildlife
Cool & Shady
Secluded
Historic

FACILITIES
Restrooms
Picnic Tables
Water

the pier, tiptoeing over narrow Arroyo del Puerto Creek at 0.10 mile. ►2 The beach begins to narrow at the 0.25-mile mark, and, at 0.5 mile, ►3 a spur to the east crawls up the eroded bluff. From the top, you can look down to the beach to the west and the historic Sebastian General Store to the east.

Continue north to a dirt access road ►4 that heads west to San Simeon Point. Along the way, clearings in the trees offer panoramic views of the coast. At the 1.0-mile mark, the trail looks down to untouched tide pools, a small rock cave, and additional rock formations. You'll reach the end of the peninsula in 1.2 miles, ►5 and there you'll find awesome views of the North Coast and the unspoiled coastline leading up to Piedras Blancas. The trail curves to the north again, heading down a dark path lined with cypress and cedar trees. The path peters out at 1.25 miles. Return the way you came.

Notice

During the summer months, you can rent a kayak at a stand on the north side of the pier. The waves at the cove are usually calmer, making this a good place for novice paddlers.

A license is not required to fish off the public pier, although Department of Fish and Game regulations and limits are enforced (see www.fgc. ca.gov/html/regs.html). Main catches off the pier are

🚶	MILESTONES	
►1	0.00	Head north from the pier.
►2	0.10	Cross Arroyo del Puerto Creek and continue up beach.
►3	0.50	Follow spur to bluff top.
►4	0.70	Path joins west-running access road.
►5	1.25	Reach the turnaround at San Simeon Point.

surfperch and jacksmelt; there is a cleaning station
located near the beginning of the pier.

Coastal Discovery Center

In July 2006, the NOAA Monterey Bay National Marine Sanctuary
and California State Parks opened the Coastal Discovery Center
(open weekends from 10 a.m. to 4 p.m) at Hearst Memorial State
Beach. The center, staffed by trained volunteers, features a handful
of marine exhibits that highlight the connection between the land
and sea.

The Monterey Bay National Marine Sanctuary stretches along
276 miles of Central California and encompasses more than 5,300
square miles of ocean. The sanctuary supports one of the world's
most diverse ecosystems, including 33 marine mammals species, 94
seabirds species, 345 fish species, and thousands of marine invertebrates and plants.

Hearst Castle

A trip up the San Simeon coast wouldn't be complete without
a stop at "the Enchanted Hill," one of the most visited places in
California. Hearst Castle, once the hilltop escape of media giant
William Randolph Hearst, offers unrivaled views of the San Simeon
coast from its perch atop the Santa Lucia Mountains. The 165-room,
127-acre castle, a modern-day museum stuffed with Hearst's collec-
tion of fine European art, was dreamed up by Hearst and translated
into reality by architect Julia Morgan. Work began on Hearst's San
Simeon retreat in 1919 and continued for almost 30 years.

Guests who once stayed there included Winston Churchill,
Charlie Chaplin, and Amelia Earhart. The Hearst Corporation
donated the castle to the state in 1958, establishing it as the Hearst
San Simeon State Historic Monument. Today, there are five guided
tours of the castle grounds. Tour 1 is the most popular, heading
through a guesthouse, the first floor of the main house, and the two
swimming pools. Other tours visit the main house's upper floors and
north wing, and the garden and guesthouse. Call (800) 444-4445 for
information or to make reservations.

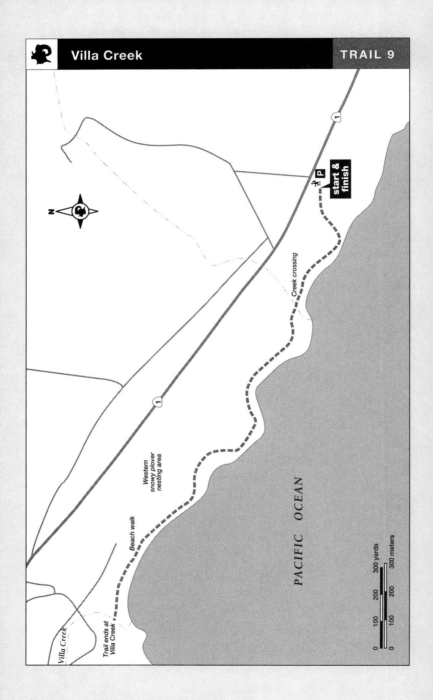

Villa Creek

TRAIL 9

N

1

1

start & finish

P

Creek crossing

Western snowy plover nesting area

Beach walk

Villa Creek

Trail ends at Villa Creek

PACIFIC OCEAN

0   100   200   300 yards

0   100   200   300 meters

Villa Creek

Villa Creek is located just north of Cayucos, tucked away in a northern crook of Estero Bay—named by Cabrillo in 1542 during his exploration of the California coast. The mouth of the creek, which creates an inviting cove that is somewhat sheltered from the ragged conditions to the north, was a popular camping spot for many explorers over the years, including Don Gaspar de Portola, who camped here in 1769. Rocks of the Franciscan Formation can be seen north of the creek, formed by volcanic activity many years ago.

Best Time

This is a great year-round hike. Because the coast can be blanketed by a marine layer throughout the year, bring a sweatshirt.

Finding the Trail

From Hwy. 1 in San Luis Obispo, head north for 15 miles to Cayucos. Continue past the exit to Cayucos Pier and drive 2.9 miles to a small paved driveway on the left-hand side that marks the trailhead to the Villa Creek Trail. The trailhead is tricky to find; it is immediately after Water Tank Hill, which can be seen on the left and recognized by the small water tank at its peak. The trailhead is midway between San Geronimo Road to the south and Villa Creek Road to the north. It is marked, alongside a gate with a State Park Boundary marker that reads NO BIKES, HORSES, OR DOGS.

TRAIL USE
Hike, Run

LENGTH
2.4 miles, 1.5 hours

VERTICAL FEET
±30

DIFFICULTY
– 1 **2** 3 4 5 +

TRAIL TYPE
Out & Back

SURFACE TYPE
Dirt

FEATURES
Beach
Birds
Tide Pools
Wildflowers
Wildlife
Great Views
Photo Opportunity
Secluded

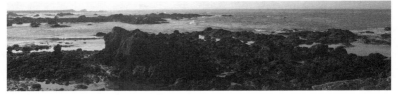

Tide pools *become most visible during a negative tide.*

Trail Description

Pass the gate, following the paved driveway ►1 out to the bluff-top trail running north to the cove at the mouth of Villa Creek. You'll reach the cliff's edge at 0.12 mile, ►2 where you'll peer all the way to Point Estero and China Harbor to the west and Cayucos Point to the south. Follow the bluff trail north toward Point Estero, hiking carefully when the single track runs up alongside the edge of the cliff. At 0.3 mile, ►3 the trail drifts away from the cliffs and crosses an intermittent stream. Watch for poison oak as the trail dips in and out of this small crevice. The trail juts back out to a nice overlook point at 0.6 mile, giving the hiker a better view of Estero Bay, which encompasses Cayucos and Morro Bay to the south.

Depending on the time of year, the latter portions of the trail may run alongside roped-off sections of the coast that are closed to the public to protect the habitat of the threatened **western snowy plover**. The habitat runs alongside the trail up to just before the 1.0-mile mark, where the trail winds down to the sandy cove. ►4 The rest of the hike is really a stroll on the **beach**, moving north to the mouth of the creek and rocky shoreline of Point Estero. Because the beach is secluded, the cove is a fun spot to soak in the sun or explore the tide pools at the north and south ends of the inlet.

Villa Creek, which originates in the Santa Lucia Mountains and parallels Villa Creek Road down to the coast, is at 1.2 miles. ►5 After reaching the creek

Birds

Beach

Stream

and taking note of the volcanic rock formations that lead to Point Estero, return to the parking area via the path you came on.

Notice

The final 0.25 mile of this hike offers access to tide pools filled with sea life. Wildlife officials discourage hikers from removing rocks, shells, or sea life from the tide zone, as many of the species that are found there are threatened. Hikers can see a handful of rare species along this stretch of coastline, including the endangered brown pelican, the threatened western snowy plover, the threatened southern sea otter, and the recently delisted peregrine falcon.

MILESTONES

▶1   0.00   Pass by the gate located near the parking area.

▶2   0.12   Trail runs along the cliff.

▶3   0.30   Drop down to an intermittent stream.

▶4   1.00   Reach the beach and continue north.

▶5   1.20   Mouth of Villa Creek marks the turnaround.

The Western Snowy Plover

NOTES

The nesting season of the western snowy plover, federally listed as a threatened species and a species of special concern in California, typically runs from March 1 through the end of September, closing portions of some San Luis Obispo County beaches. State park managers usually install boundary fencing and signs to warn the public to stay out of dune areas where the birds nest.

The tiny shorebird is a 6- to 7-inch, sand-colored species with a black mark on each side of the breast, behind each eye, and on the brow. While its habitat is closed to the public for much of the year, this particular trail runs close enough to the birds that they can been seen in full detail with a decent set of binoculars.

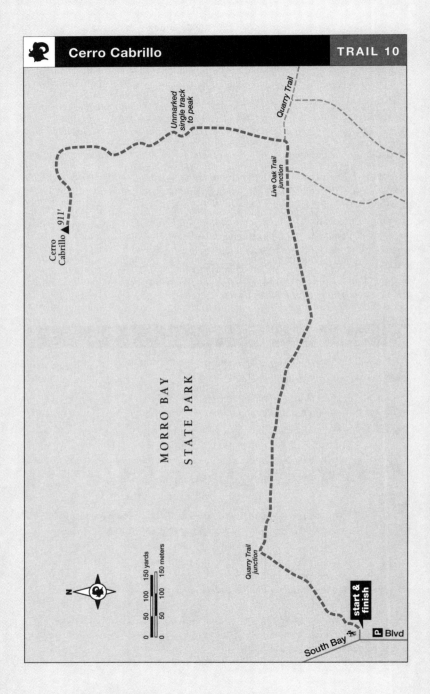

Cerro Cabrillo

TRAIL 10

MORRO BAY
STATE PARK

Cerro
Cabrillo ▲ 911'

Unmarked
single track
to peak

Quarry Trail

Live Oak Trail
junction

Quarry Trail
junction

start &
finish

South Bay
P Blvd

N

0   50   100   150 yards
0   50   100   150 meters

Cerro Cabrillo

Cerro Cabrillo is one of the most popular of the Nine Sisters because it lies between two of the region's most impressive volcanic plugs, Morro Rock and Hollister Peak, both of which are closed to public climbing or hiking of any kind. Instead, Morro Bay trailblazers are left with 665-foot Black Hill and 911-foot Cerro Cabrillo, the latter of which offers the area's best views of the estuary, coastline, and remaining chain of Sisters.

Diarist Juan Crespi, who stumbled upon the butte along with Don Gaspar de Portola during their Spanish land expedition from San Diego to Monterey Bay in the late 1760s, best described the view from Cerro Cabrillo: "An estuary of immense size enters the valley, so large that it looks like a harbor to us," he wrote on September 8, 1769. "Its mouth opens to the southwest. ... To the north, we saw a great rock [Morro Rock] in the form of a morro, which at high tide is isolated from the coast by little less than a gunshot." While Morro Rock is no longer isolated from the mainland, the view is still pretty much the same from Cabrillo Peak, with the exception of a few boats, houses, business buildings, a golf course, and the three smokestacks.

TRAIL USE
Hike, Run, Bike, Horse
LENGTH
2.5 miles, 1.5 hours
VERTICAL FEET
±900
DIFFICULTY
– 1 2 3 **4** 5 +
TRAIL TYPE
Out & Back
SURFACE TYPE
Dirt

FEATURES
Mountain
Steep
Birds
Wildflowers
Wildlife
Great Views
Photo Opportunity
Secluded
Geologic

Best Time

The hike to the top of Cerro Cabrillo, named after Portuguese explorer Juan Cabrillo, is at its best in the summer and fall, as the climb becomes difficult during the wet season. Like from most of the region's coastal trails, the views on this hike are best on clear, sunny days, which can be few and far in between in

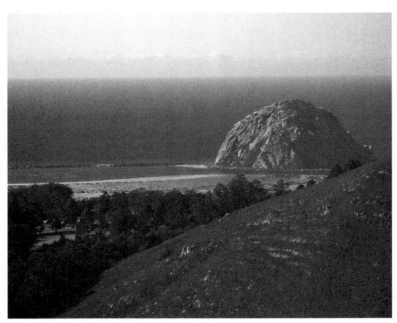

Distant Morro Rock and Black Hill, *in the foreground, are part of the Nine Sisters.*

Morro Bay. Take note of any warnings posted at the trailhead kiosk about poison oak, ticks, or mountain lions, and try to hike with a partner.

Finding the Trail

From Hwy. 1 in south Morro Bay, take the South Bay Blvd. exit toward Los Osos for 1.5 miles. The dirt parking lot is on the left.

Trail Description

From the trailhead kiosk, ▶1 follow the dirt single track that meets up with the Quarry Trail. The Chumash Trail branches off the main track at 0.2 mile, so stay to the right. At 0.5 mile, you'll pass the

Live Oak Trail to the right; stay straight and follow the Quarry Trail to 0.8 mile, where an unmarked single track ►2 veers off to the left and makes the **steep climb** to the peak. The trail, which winds through deerweed, soap plant, and mallow, is tough to miss in the summer and early fall, but may be overgrown with grass and wildflowers during the spring.

 Steep

San Luis Obispo County's Nine Sisters are a chain of volcanic peaks between Morro Bay and San Luis Obispo.

You'll know you've passed the Cabrillo Peak Trail if you've reached the beginning of the Ridge Park or Cenet trails. This is where the trail really starts to climb. At the 1.0-mile mark, ►3 Hollister Peak towers to the east, and the bay and Morro Rock are to the west. This is the most challenging portion of the trail, reaching 825 feet by 1.2 miles and requiring hikers to tackle some small boulders on the way to the top. From the peak, ►4 on a clear day, you can see from Montaña de Oro all the way up to the Cayucos coast. The estuary is a **spectacular sight** from 911 feet above, with its maze-like channels and fingers that stretch all the way from Morro Bay State Park all the way to Montaña de Oro State Park. Morro Rock can be seen on the other side of Black Hill, another one of the Sisters located next to the golf course. To return to the parking lot, retrace your steps, descending the steep portions of the trail slowly to avoid slipping. ►5

 Great Views

A Closer Look at the Estuary

OPTIONS

Impressed with the views of the Morro Bay Estuary but want to get a closer look? Kayak Horizons (805-772-6444) on the Embarcadero has kayak rentals and on weekends even offers guided kayak tours of the bay and the back portions of the estuary. While paddling around the bay, you'll get up close and personal with hundreds of types of birds that make this sanctuary home, including the peregrine falcon and the endangered brown pelican.

Notice

Mountain bikes and horses are allowed on this and most Morro Bay State Park trails, although this steep single track to the peak is aimed at hikers who aren't afraid to boulder hop at the top. Bikers and riders would be better suited to stick with the Quarry, Ridge Park, or Cenet trails. Remember to tuck in your shoelaces when boulder hopping on hikes.

🚶 MILESTONES

▶1	0.00	Start your climb at the kiosk and stay straight, passing the Live Oak trailhead.
▶2	0.80	Veer off the Quarry Trail to the single track on the left, which makes the climb to the peak.
▶3	1.00	Views of Hollister Peak to the east and Morro Rock to the west.
▶4	1.50	The peak can be reached with some climbing to 911 feet.
▶5	1.75	Return the way you came, using caution on the way down from the peak.

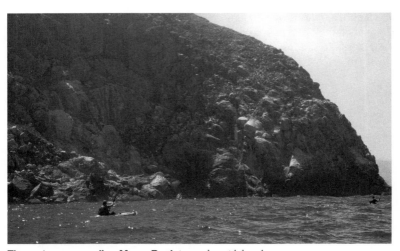

The water surrounding Morro Rock *is popular with kayakers.*

Additional Trails

OPTIONS

The Cerro Cabrillo area has a handful of other self-explanatory, out-and-back trails that are popular with hikers and riders:

- The Quarry Trail is a 2.0-mile hike that passes through several sites that were once quarried for rock. Much of the rock was used to create Hwy. 1.

- Other old quarry sites can be found along the Chumash Trail, which begins near the main trailhead and wraps around the opposite side of the mountain and parallels South Bay Blvd.

- The trail up to Chorro Hill passes Turtle Rock, a 210-foot outcropping at the northwest base of the plug.

- The Live Oak Trail, 0.5 mile into the Quarry Trail, heads to 330-foot Portola Point and offers lower-elevation views of the estuary, which is a protected bird sanctuary and favorite getaway for bird-watchers.

- The Cenet Trail is a popular run for mountain bikers and riders on horseback, while the Ridge Park Trail is popular with climbers.

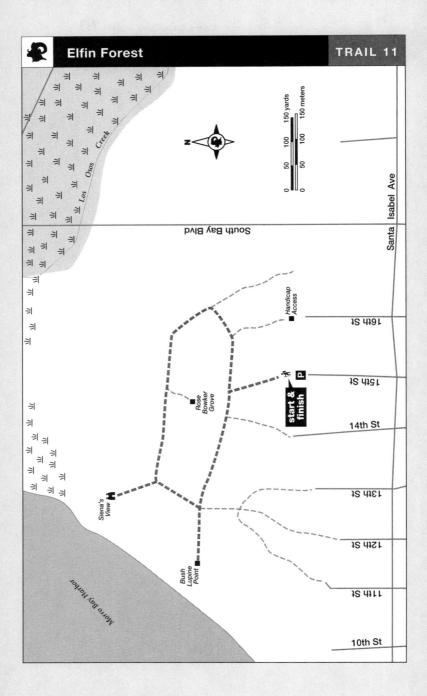

Los Osos Creek

South Bay Blvd

Santa Isabel Ave

N

0   50   100   150 yards
0   50   100   150 meters

Handicap
Access

16th St

15th St

start &
finish

14th St

Rose
Bowker
Grove

Siena's
View

13th St

12th St

Bush
Lupine
Point

11th St

Morro Bay Harbor

10th St

Elfin Forest

This boardwalk trail loops around the 90-acre Elfin Forest Natural Area at the southeast end of the Morro Bay where Los Osos Creek dumps into the estuary near Los Osos/Baywood Park. In just 1.0 mile, the trail goes over coastal dune scrub, maritime chaparral, and pygmy oak woodland, all while offering some of the best views around of the estuary. Because this is a wheelchair-accessible boardwalk, it is fit for hikers of all ages and abilities, including parents, their children, and strollers. The west side of the loop has a pair of lookouts that are perfect for birding, as the estuary is home to hundreds of species each year.

Best Time

The trail is open all year. Workdays are held on the first Saturday of the month. Guided nature walks take place on the third Saturday of the month. See the trail guide brochures located near the 16th St. entrance for additional information on walks and workdays. Check tide tables to see how high or low the tide will be during your hike. If you want to see the estuary's maze-like waterways, wait until low tide. If you want to look out over a full bay, wait until high tide.

Finding the Trail

From San Luis Obispo, drive north on Hwy. 1 for 13 miles to the Los Osos/Baywood Park exit. Make a left on South Bay Blvd., traveling 2.4 miles to Santa Ysabel Ave. Make a right, followed by another right

TRAIL USE
Hike, Run, Bike, Horse
LENGTH
1.0 mile, 1.0 hour
VERTICAL FEET
±80
DIFFICULTY
− **1** 2 3 4 5 +
TRAIL TYPE
Loop
SURFACE TYPE
Mixed

FEATURES
Handicap Access
Child Friendly
Dogs Allowed
Wetland
Birds
Wildlife
Great Views
Photo Opportunity

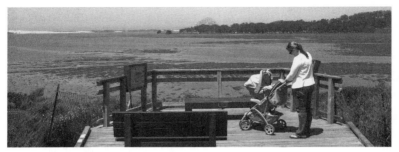

The boardwalk offers up-close views *of the estuary and Morro Bay harbor.*

The "pygmy oaks" are more than 100 years old, and limited to about 12 feet in height because of the coastal dune environment.

 Handicap Access

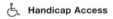 Great Views

on 15th St., and drive to the end of the road, parking in the dirt spaces on either side of the road near the trailhead. Do not block driveways, and respect private property. There is wheelchair access at the 16th St. entrance.

Trail Description

The trail starts in the dunes and passes over the sand for 50 feet ►1 to the boardwalk. Follow the steps up to the boardwalk and take the **wooden walkway** to the right, passing counterclockwise around the path. ►2 The path meets the 16th St. entrance at 0.11 mile. A trail-guide brochure can be picked up where the 16th St. entrance meets the main boardwalk. There are more than a dozen benches along the loop, including one near the 16th St. entrance.

The trail passes another entrance via 17th St. before making a sharp turn to the left where the path overlooks the estuary to the right and Evan's and Rose Bowker groves to the left. At 0.3 mile, a spur to the left leads to Rose Bowker Grove, ►3 where stunted coast live oaks grow.

Continue down the path and stay right at a fork in trail. This portion of the boardwalk leads to Siena's View, ►4 one of two lookout points where you can **gaze out over the estuary**. Siena's View marks the halfway point of the walk, at 0.5 mile.

The viewpoint overlooks the murky waterways below; the estuary's many channels can be seen best during a negative tide. Morro Rock marks the mouth of the bay to the north, kicking off a chain of morros that includes Black Hill and Cerro Cabrillo, visible to the northeast.

Return to the main boardwalk and head right, toward Bush Lupine Point. ►5 The path to the second lookout is on the right at 0.64 mile. The Bush Lupine Point, at 0.7 mile, has a higher vantage point over the estuary and the sandpit to the west, and is a great perch for **bird-watchers** charting the hundreds of bird species that visit the bay.

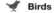 **Birds**

Retrace your steps to the main walk and continue east to the 15th St. entrance, ►6 passing similar spurs from 11th, 12th, and 13th streets. The stairs back to 15th St. are at 0.91 mile, and the parking area is within 0.1 mile.

Notice

Trail users are encouraged to remain on the boardwalk to minimize erosion and damage to the native plant species.

🚶	**MILESTONES**	
►1	0.00	Cross the dunes for 50 feet to the boardwalk.
►2	0.11	Follow the boardwalk in a counterclockwise fashion.
►3	0.30	The boardwalk passes Rose Bowker Grove on the left.
►4	0.40	Stay right at the fork to Siena's View.
►5	0.60	Continuing down the main boardwalk; stay right at the next fork to Bush Lupine Point.
►6	0.80	Head back to the main boardwalk and continue straight to the 15th St. entrance, making a right and following the sandy single track back to the car.

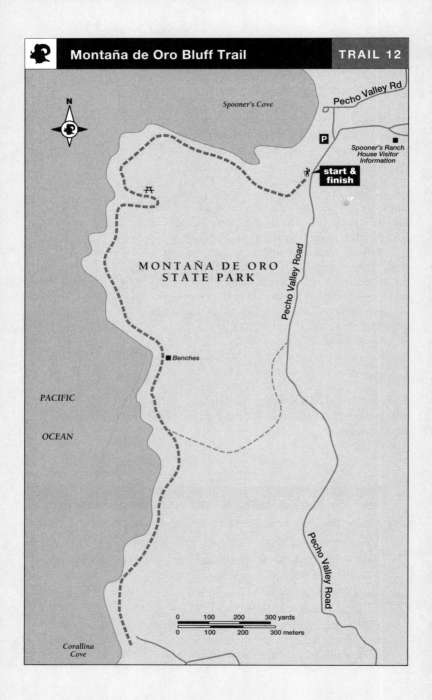

Montaña de Oro Bluff Trail

TRAIL 12

N

Spooner's Cove

Pecho Valley Rd

P

Spooner's Ranch House Visitor Information

start & finish

M O N T A Ñ A   D E   O R O
S T A T E   P A R K

Pecho Valley Road

■ *Benches*

PACIFIC

OCEAN

| 0 | 100 | 200 | 300 yards |
| 0 | 100 | 200 | 300 meters |

Pecho Valley Road

Corallina Cove

Montaña de Oro Bluff Trail

If this bluff-top trail isn't the finest on the Central Coast, it's certainly a close second. And like many of the gorgeous trails in the region, this well-groomed and relatively flat run gets plenty of action on the weekends. Jogger, hikers, mountain bikers, kids, parents, grandparents—this trail sees it all. As its name describes, the dirt trail runs along the top of Montaña de Oro State Park's shale and sediment bluffs, which jut into the pounding surf to create spectacular rock outcroppings and saltwater scenes that rival the views of any coastal trail this side of Big Sur.

Best Time

Because the trail is well maintained, it is a fun, easy hike all year. Most of the hiking pressure on this trail occurs on weekends and during the afternoons and early evenings during the week. Hike with caution along portions of the trail that run along shale cliffs and stay clear of the steep drop-offs during wet conditions or high surf advisories.

Finding the Trail

From Hwy. 101 in southern San Luis Obispo, take the Los Osos Valley Road exit west for 11.5 miles to Los Osos. Los Osos Valley Road becomes Pecho Valley Road near Montaña de Oro State Park. From the park entrance, travel 5.0 miles past the campground and park in the dirt turnout on the right just after the larger parking area at Spooner's Cove. The Bluff Trail is clearly signed at the end of the turnoff

TRAIL USE
Hike, Run, Bike

LENGTH
3.3 miles, 1.5 hours

VERTICAL FEET
±80

DIFFICULTY
– 1 **2** 3 4 5 +

TRAIL TYPE
Out & Back

SURFACE TYPE
Dirt

FEATURES
Child Friendly
Steep
Beach
Tide Pools
Wildflowers
Great Views
Geologic

FACILITIES
Restrooms
Picnic Tables
Water
Phone
Campground

Great Views

 Tide Pools

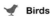 **Birds**

south of Spooner's Cove. Trail maps and brochures on the state park can be picked up at the ranger station across the road, near the campground.

Trail Description

From the trailhead atop the bluffs south of Spooner's Cove, cross the small bridge ►1 over a seasonal creek and head toward the ocean. At 0.38 mile, the trail turns left as it runs into the first shale cliff, ►2 which drops off to a secluded cove below, which is accessible via Spooner's Cove. This overlook, also known as Islay Point, looks back on Spooner's Cove and offers a **breathtaking backdrop** made up of Morro Rock, Morro Dunes Natural Preserve, jetties, and the bay to the north.

A couple of spurs lead off the trail to the right at 0.4 mile. ►3 They wind down to the rocky beach, and can be fun side trips **during a low tide** if surf conditions are calm. If you must venture down to the beach, be sure to follow designated trails only and use extreme caution on the descent.

The trail crosses another bridge at 0.6 mile. ►4 Continue straight, down the hard-packed dirt trail, staying to the right of oncoming pedestrians. At the 1.0-mile mark, ►5 the trail drops down to another point that extends into the ocean. A picnic table is located on a small patch of grass at the rear of a quaint cove. The table is a popular resting point and lunchtime getaway for folks in the Los Osos/ Baywood Park area. Take a breather here, listening to the crashing waves and the **various sea birds** that flock about. Keep an eye out for brown pelicans and snowy plovers, a pair of rare species that call this stretch of the coastline home. You may also see peregrine falcons, which are also infrequently sighted.

Follow the trail south, watching your step at the 1.35-mile mark as the trail runs right alongside the cliff, a good 20 or 30 feet above an interesting set of

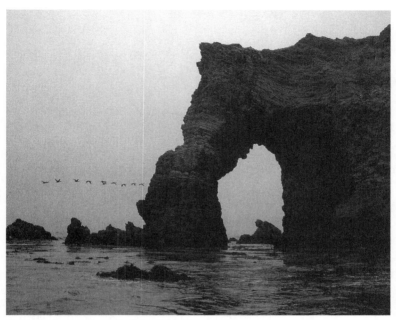

Point Buchon, *to the south off the Diablo Canyon coast*

rock outcroppings. Take a good look at the tallest of the rock formations, which has been hollowed by the surf over time to create a small archway.

A **V**-shaped set of benches constructed by a local Eagle Scout troop offers another resting point at 1.55 miles, ▶6 along with nice views of the off-limits coastline located to the south on Diablo Canyon property. The trail continues, offering a glimpse of Grotto Rock, and finally comes to a dead end at a barbed wire fence, at 1.66 miles. This fence marks Diablo Canyon property and is the turnaround. ▶7 From the fence line, take a last glimpse out to Point Buchon and the remote cove where Coon Creek washes into the Pacific. Trail users can follow the spur to the left, toward the Coon Creek trailhead parking lot, and follow paved Pecho Valley Road in a

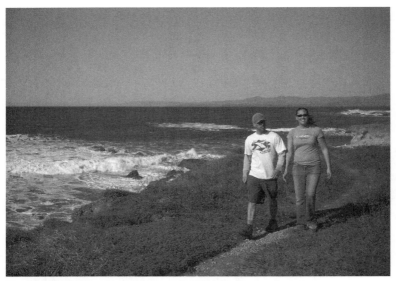

The Bluff Trail *runs right along the rugged cliffs leading down to the surf.*

loop-like fashion back to the car. Most hikers return the way they came because of the can't-miss views along the way.

🚶 MILESTONES

▶1	0.00	Start at the signed trailhead and cross a small bridge.
▶2	0.38	Trail curves to the left, offering views of Spooner's Cove.
▶3	0.40	Stay straight past the spurs to the right, which go down to the beach.
▶4	0.60	Continue over another bridge, which clears a seasonal stream.
▶5	1.00	The first of two benches offers a resting area to the right.
▶6	1.55	A second set of benches is on the left.
▶7	1.66	Trail ends at a barbed-wire fence, which marks the turnaround.

Other Trails

Because Montaña de Oro State Park encompasses more than 8,000 square miles, including 7.0 miles of shoreline, it's tough to pick an additional trail to take while you're there. The good thing about all of the other trails in the area is they rarely see as much pressure as the famed Bluff Trail—keep in mind more than a half-million people visit the park each year, according to park officials. Aside from the Bluff Trail, the Sand Spit and Hazard Canyon Reef trails are probably the most popular. Both trails are in the northern part of the park, on the west side of Pecho Valley Road.

The Sand Spit Day Use Area is accessible via Sand Spit Road, which is your first right after entering the park. The boardwalk hike down to the beach is less than 0.5 mile, but you could extend the trail with a beach walk to the north. You can tack another 8 or 9 miles (round trip) onto the hike if you walk all the way up to the Morro Bay inlet. From the harbor mouth, you'll have a tremendous view of the southern face of Morro Rock, where peregrine falcons have been known to reside.

The parking area at Hazard Canyon is south of the Sand Spit turnoff, on the west side of Pecho Valley Road at a clearing in the tall eucalyptus trees. The short hike down to Hazard Canyon is less than a mile, but hikers can add a couple of miles by heading south along the beach or on the out-and-back Dune Trail.

During the production of this book, a 1.0-mile loop to Point Buchon opened to the public. The trailhead for this trail is located at the parking area for the Coon Creek Trail.

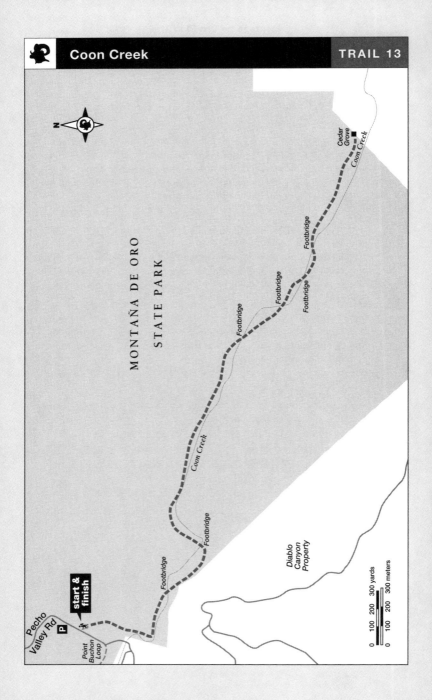

TRAIL 13

Coon Creek

N

MONTAÑA DE ORO
STATE PARK

Cedar
Grove

Coon Creek

Footbridge

Footbridge

Footbridge

Footbridge

Footbridge

Coon Creek

Footbridge

Footbridge

Footbridge

start &
finish

Pecho
Valley Rd

P

Point
Buchon Loop

Diablo
Canyon
Property

0   100 200 300 yards

0   100 200 300 meters

Coon Creek

Coon Creek, likely named for the many raccoons that inhabit the area, originates 1,300 feet above sea level near Irish Hills and tumbles past Ruda Canyon and Montaña de Oro State Park before dumping into the Pacific just north of Point Buchon. This creekside trail runs along the southern perimeter of the park, weaving through riparian habitat and numerous groves of oak, willow, maple, pine, and cottonwood. The single track follows the creek upstream, crosses its narrow flows via a handful of wooden footbridges, and ends at an old cabin site and cedar grove.

TRAIL USE
Hike, Run
LENGTH
4.4 miles, 2.0 hours
VERTICAL FEET
±250
DIFFICULTY
– 1 2 **3** 4 5 +
TRAIL TYPE
Out & Back
SURFACE TYPE
Dirt

Best Time

The park's name, which means "Mountain of Gold," comes from the golden wildflowers that bloom here in the spring—which is the most scenic time of year to hike Coon Creek. Because of the mild temperatures along the coast and the shady trees that line the latter half of the trail, the trail is also a good summer alternative when the fog spoils the view of the bluff trails nearby.

FEATURES
Stream
Fall Color
Birds
Wildflowers
Wildlife
Cool & Shady
Camping
Geologic

FACILITIES
Restrooms
Picnic Tables
Campground
Visitors Center

Finding the Trail

From Hwy. 101 in southern San Luis Obispo, take the Los Osos Valley Road exit west for 11.5 miles to Los Osos. Los Osos Valley Road becomes Pecho Valley Road near Montaña de Oro State Park. From the park entrance, travel 6.2 miles past the campground and Spooner's Cove to the parking area at the end of the road. The Coon Creek trailhead is

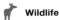 **Wildlife**

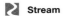 **Stream**

clearly signed at the end of the parking lot. A trail map is available for $1 at the visitors center and is worth picking up, considering the park is packed with trails and there is no parking fee for day use.

Trail Description

The trail starts out at the parking lot, where Pecho Valley Road dead-ends to the public about 1.2 miles south of the campground and headquarters. The single track passes a picnic table ►1 that is popular with the **resident raccoons**, which can often be seen during the morning and evening hours. Park rangers encourage hikers to stay away from the raccoons and avoid feeding them.

The first footbridge crossing the year-round creek is within the first 0.1 mile. You'll come to two more bridges within the first mile, including crossings at 0.4 mile and 0.62 mile. ►2 A canopy of willow, oak and maple provides plenty of shade where the trail borders the creek. The trail pulls away from the **creek** and the shade a bit after the first mile, passing a junction to the Rattlesnake Flats Trail (3.2 miles) on the left-hand side at 1.03 miles. ►3

Stay straight, following the creek upstream to a fourth footbridge, at 1.27 miles. ►4 Look down to the tiny pools below for a chance to see wild steelhead trout, which often swim up Coon Creek from the Pacific to spawn. A fifth and sixth bridge are located at 1.4 miles and 1.5 miles. The second half of the trail dips back into a shady canopy whose gnarled branches are camouflaged by Spanish moss. Watch your head as you pass by the low-hanging limbs at the 1.5-mile mark.

The final footbridge is at 1.7 miles. ►5 Cross the bridge and head past the spur to the Oats Peak Trail (4.8 miles) at the 2.0-mile mark. The end is near, 0.2 mile ahead, at the cedar grove.

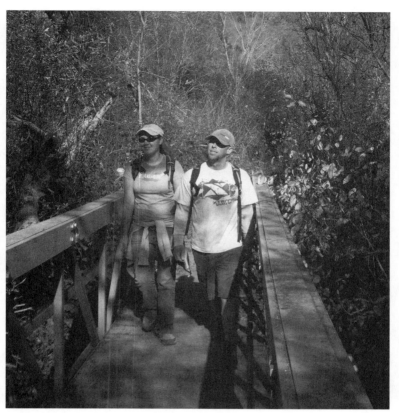

A footbridge *across a creek filled with darting steelhead*

The cedar grove is the turnaround ▶6 and **a great place to get out of the sun** and take a breather or have a picnic in the clearing where an old hunting cabin once stood, between the downed trees. The creek continues to the southeast, but the trail is not maintained past the old cabin site, and poison oak litters the unmarked game trail that follows the creek. Return the way you came, or hike back to Pecho Valley Road via the Oats Peak Trail or the Rattlesnake Flats Trail.

Cool & Shady

Notice

There is a drive-in campground with about 50 campsites near the Spooner Ranch House and campground headquarters. A few hike-in sites also are available via the Rattlesnake Flats, Badger, Reservoir Flats, and Bloody Nose trails, and there is a horse camp off Hazard Canyon Road. Call (800) 444-7275 for more information.

The Diablo Canyon Power Plant is 2.4 miles south of the Coon Creek Trail's turnaround. The nuclear power plant provides electricity for more than 1.6 million homes in California. The plant is surrounded by 12,000 acres that an area mostly off-limits to the public because of security concerns. If you hear sirens blaring at the park, tune in to 1400 AM or 98.1 FM for emergency information.

𝍐 MILESTONES

▶1   0.00   Head toward the creek, passing a picnic area.

▶2   0.62   Three footbridges span the creek in first mile.

▶3   1.03   Continue past a spur, toward Rattlesnake Flats.

▶4   1.27   Pass three more bridges over the next 0.25 mile.

▶5   1.70   Cross over the final bridge.

▶6   2.20   Cedar grove marks the turnaround.

Two Adjacent Trails

There are two main trails that connect with the Coon Creek Trail and return to Pecho Valley Road. The Rattlesnake Flats Trail (3.2 miles) is accessible just over 1.0 mile into the Coon Creek Trail, while the Oats Peak Trail (4.8 miles) is accessible at the 2.0-mile mark.

Rattlesnake Flats is a popular trail because of the environmental campsite, located about 2.0 miles from the junction with Coon Creek. The trail eventually meets with the Badger Trail, after 3.0 miles, and spits out at Pecho Valley Road. After reaching Pecho Valley Road, you'll have to hike another 0.5 mile south to the parking area.

The Oats Peak Trail is a grueling climb to a peak that rises to an elevation of 1,373 feet. Next to Valencia Peak (1,347 feet), this summit offers the best vista point overlooking the southern portion of the park. From Oats Peak, the trail heads east for a couple of miles to Alan Peak (1,649 feet) and west, back to the park headquarters—which makes it a better point-to-point hike if you leave one vehicle near Spooner's Cove. You could also return to the Coon Creek parking area by taking Pecho Valley Road south for 1.2 miles, which would make for a 7.0-mile trek.

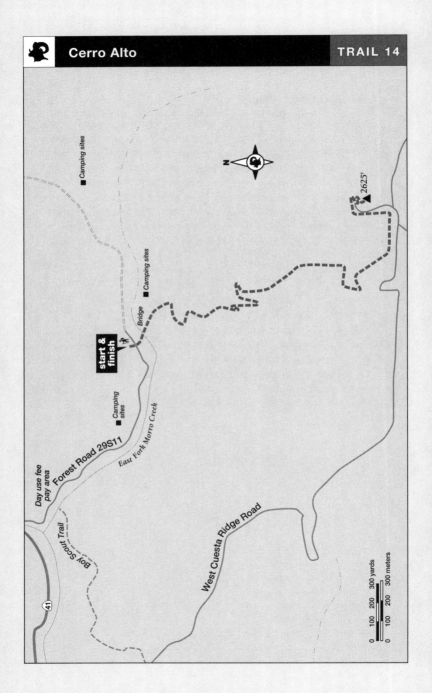

Cerro Alto

TRAIL 14

2625'

Camping sites

Camping sites

Bridge

start & finish

Camping sites

East Fork Morro Creek

Forest Road 29S11

Day use fee pay area

Boy Scout Trail

West Cuesta Ridge Road

41

0   100   200   300 yards
0   100   200   300 meters

Cerro Alto

Cerro Alto is a steep climb but is worth the journey for its amazing roundabout views of San Luis Obispo County. From the boulders atop the peak, you'll see awe-inspiring scenes, including the Estero Bay coast, North County, San Luis Obispo, and all the magnificent morros in between. This multiuse trail, halfway between Morro Bay and Atascadero, is one of the few in the inland North County region that is open to mountain bikers, dog walkers, and horseback riders.

Best Time

Because the trail climbs to 2,600 feet and has very little shade along the way, this hike is at its best in the morning or in the cooler months. Also, it's a good idea to choose a clear day to hike, as the coastal fog can put a damper on the views at the top. If you go in the summer, be sure to get an early start as there is very little shade after the first 0.5 mile.

Finding the Trail

From Hwy. 1 in Morro Bay, take the Hwy. 41 exit toward Atascadero. Follow Hwy. 41 for 7.0 miles until you see signs for the campground on the right at forest road 29S11. Alternatively, from Hwy. 101 in Atascadero, take Hwy. 41 west toward Morro Bay for about 9.0 miles and make a left at 29S11. Pay the $5 entry free at the kiosk and continue down the road for about a mile to the day-use area south of the campsite host. The trailhead is between campsites 15 and 16, near the footbridge over the East Fork of Morro Creek.

TRAIL USE
Hike, Run, Bike, Horse
LENGTH
4.0 miles, 2.0 hours
VERTICAL FEET
±1604
DIFFICULTY
– 1 2 3 **4 5** +
TRAIL TYPE
Out & Back
SURFACE TYPE
Dirt

FEATURES
Parking Fee
Dogs Allowed
Canyon
Mountain
Stream
Birds
Great Views

FACILITIES
Restrooms
Picnic Tables
Water
Campground

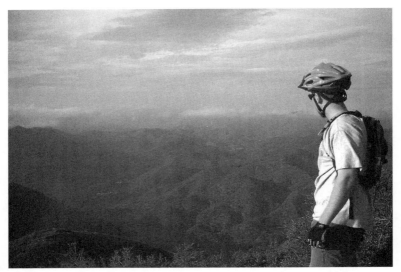

The later stages of the Cerro Alto Trail *can be a tough climb for mountain bikers.*

Trail Description

 Steep

Head over the bridge ▶1 that crosses the East Fork of Morro Creek and start your 2.0-mile climb up to the summit. At 0.4 mile, you will already have **climbed 275 feet** and will be looking down on the campground and on the highway ▶2 that bridges the gap between the coast and inland North County. This is a good perch for bird-watchers looking for the predatory hawks and turkey vultures that circle above. The occasional banana slug also can be seen at the lower elevations of the trail in the early spring.

By the 0.7-mile mark, the trail really starts to climb. Stay left on the trail marked by the SUMMIT sign ▶3 and continue winding your way up the mountain. At just under 0.1 mile, you'll reach a crossroads in your journey. This is the halfway point and is a good spot for a quick breather. Stay straight on the trail ▶4 to reach the summit. Take your time from here, as you've already reached the 2,000-foot mark by 1.3 miles and can see the ocean on a clear day. Continue up the trail and you can catch glimpses of the Morro Bay, Cayucos, and San Simeon coasts, Whale Rock Reservoir, and Morro Rock. At 2.0 miles, you've finally made it to the Cerro Alto Summit, ►5 2,625 feet above sea level. To the south is the city of San Luis Obispo, beyond Cuesta Ridge. Atascadero is to the east, and Los Osos and **Morro Bay** to the west. Return to the trailhead the same way you came.

Great Views

Notice

Poison oak is common in the late spring and early summer, so if you're hiking with your dog, keep it on a short leash for the first mile of the hike.

Notice

Keep in mind this is a multiuse trail shared by mountain bikers, hikers, and equestrians, so use caution when coming around blind turns and other narrow portions of the single-track sections.

🚶		MILESTONES
►1	0.0	From the bridge crossing the creek, start heading up the trail.
►2	0.4	The campground and highway can be seen below during the climb.
►3	0.7	Stay left on the trail marked by the SUMMIT sign.
►4	0.9	At the crossroad, stay straight to reach the summit.
►5	2.0	After reaching the summit, return by the same route.

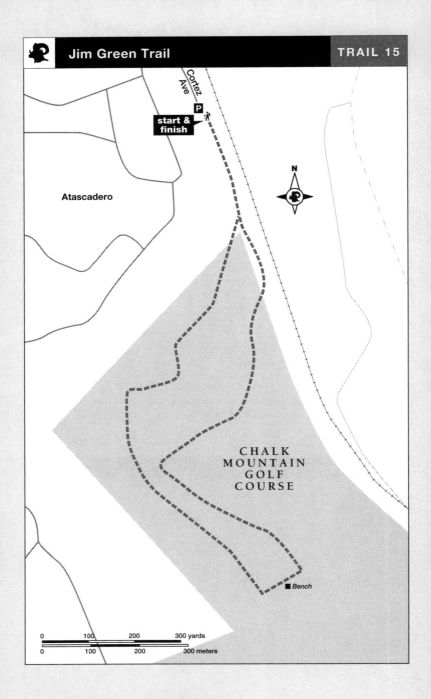

start & finish

Cortez Ave

P

N

Atascadero

CHALK
MOUNTAIN
GOLF
COURSE

■ *Bench*

| 0 | 100 | 200 | 300 yards |
| 0 | 100 | 200 | 300 meters |

Jim Green Trail

Because this single track in Atascadero is fairly wide and well groomed, it is a popular loop for triathlon-training runners and unhurried bird-watchers alike. It's also the perfect destination for a family hike in the evening or on a lazy weekend afternoon. The dirt trail wraps around towering moss-strewn oak trees and hillsides that look as if they've been painted with wildflowers each spring. The second half of the county park's trail runs alongside the Chalk Mountain Golf Course and loops back to the trailhead, which is located across the train tracks from the Salinas River.

Best Time

While much of the trail is shaded because of the large oak trees, 100°F temperatures in the summer make the loop less inviting. Hike in the mornings during the summer months.

Finding the Trail

From San Luis Obispo, take Hwy. 101 north to Atascadero and exit at Curbaril Ave. Take a right on Curbaril for 1.0 mile and take another right on Cortez Ave. just before the railroad tracks. Park in the dirt turnout at the end of the road, making sure not to block any residential driveways. The trailhead is at the end of the parking area.

TRAIL USE
Hike, Run, Bike, Horse
LENGTH
1.7 miles, 1.0 hour
VERTICAL FEET
±60
DIFFICULTY
− 1 **2** 3 4 5 +
TRAIL TYPE
Loop
SURFACE TYPE
Dirt

FEATURES
Child Friendly
Dogs Allowed
Meadow
Birds
Wildflowers
Wildlife
Great Views

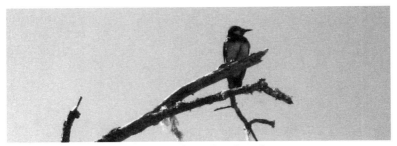

An acorn woodpecker *perched in an oak tree along the trail*

Trail Description

The trail doesn't exactly feel like a wilderness hike at the onset, but that changes after it leaves the neighborhood near the trailhead. ▶1 There is a kiosk at the start with a map of the **well-maintained loop trail**, which starts off at an elevation of 921 feet and never passes the 1,000-foot mark.

The dirt single track comes to a fork at 0.14 mile. ▶2 Stay right and follow the loop in a counterclockwise fashion. This is when the trail starts to feel like a trail again, winding through giant oak trees where Spanish moss hangs from branches like a wise man's beard, and acorn woodpeckers go a knockin' like a door-to-door salesman. There's a reason the **redheaded woodpecker** is the logo of the Chalk Mountain Golf Course. These black and white birds are everywhere.

The only notable climb of the trail comes at 0.3 mile, with the trail slowly rising to 980 feet before following a rift down toward the green fairways. The trail overlooks the golf course and a large water tank on the adjacent hillside at 0.75 mile. ▶3 A bench has been installed just before the 1.0-mile mark, ▶4 overlooking a meandering creek on the front nine, where **mule deer** often graze in the rough. From this resting point, the trail bends around to the northwest and heads back to the trailhead. You leave the vicinity of the golf course, and your path looks

Child Friendly

Birds

Wildlife

over a water treatment plant at 1.25 miles. ►5 The trail rejoins the first leg of the hike and spits back out at the parking area in less than a half mile.

Notice

This Heilmann Regional Park trail may be tucked between a small neighborhood and a golf course, but don't be surprised if you run into wildlife other than birds on this or any other Central Coast trail. The kiosk located at the trailhead cautions hikers to look out for rattlesnakes, but it says nothing of bears—that's right, bears. While bears or mountain lions rarely make their way down to public trails, a mother bear and cub were seen near this trail as recently as May 2007.

The trail is named after the late Jim Green of Atascadero, an outdoor enthusiast who was responsible for helping create a number of hiking trails in San Luis Obispo County.

MILESTONES

►1	0.00	Follow the loop in a counterclockwise fashion.
►2	0.15	Stay right at fork.
►3	0.75	Trail runs alongside the golf course.
►4	0.85	A bench offers a resting spot.
►5	1.25	Trail heads back to first leg and spits out at parking lot.

Heilmann Regional Park

OPTIONS

This park has it all—tennis courts, horseshoe pits, barbecue and picnic areas, a dog park, and an 18-hole golf course, not to mention the North County's only disc golf course.

While the Jim Green Trail is accessed via the north entrance on Cortez Ave., just about everything else the park has to offer can be reached via the main entrance on El Bordo Ave., about a mile south of El Camino Real. There is one maintained trail at this second location—the 1.3 mile Blue Oak Trail, which is open to hiking and biking only and follows a dirt path around the perimeter of the park. Watch for flying Frisbees flung from the nearby disc golf course.

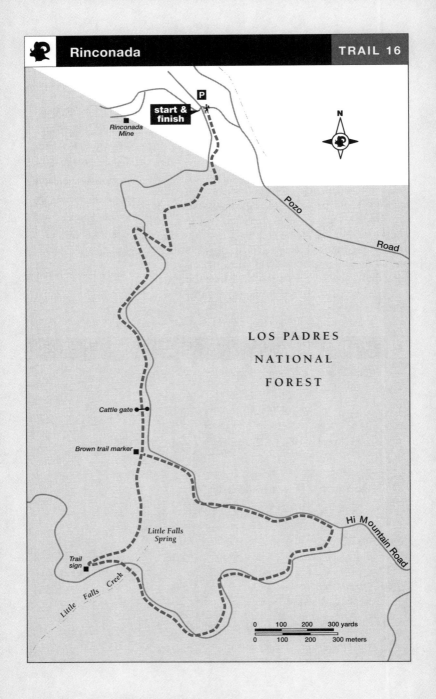

Rinconada

TRAIL 16

start & finish

P

Rinconada Mine

N

Pozo

Road

LOS PADRES

NATIONAL

FOREST

Cattle gate

Brown trail marker

Little Falls Spring

Hi Mountain Road

Trail sign

Little Falls Creek

| 0 | 100 | 200 | 300 yards |
| 0 | 100 | 200 | 300 meters |

Rinconada

The Rinconada Trail is a challenging multiuse trail tucked between Santa Margarita and Lopez lakes in the Santa Margarita foothills of the Los Padres National Forest. The trails in the area were closed to the public from 2003 to 2005 as the U.S. Environmental Protection Agency cleaned up pollutants near the old Rinconada Mine, but were up and running again by the summer of 2005.

This particular route is unique in that it is made up of a technical single track, which includes all the switchbacks and a climb of 500-plus feet in the first 1.4 miles, along with a fun downhill run on a dirt access road. The vegetation is as diverse as the trail itself, comprising a medley of flowery grasslands, chaparral shrublands, and oak woodlands.

Best Time

The trail is open all year, although it may be closed during the rainy season to prevent damage to the surface. Spring is best for the wildflowers. There is no potable water on the trail, so bring plenty, especially in the summer, when temperatures can reach triple figures.

Finding the Trail

From Hwy. 101 in San Luis Obispo, head north over the Cuesta Grade and take the Santa Margarita exit, which becomes Hwy. 58. Take the highway through town for 1.6 miles, turning right to follow it over the railroad tracks toward Santa Margarita Lake. Stay on the highway for another 1.6 miles, but stay straight

TRAIL USE
Hike, Run, Bike, Horse
LENGTH
4.6 miles, 2.5 hours
VERTICAL FEET
±718
DIFFICULTY
– 1 2 3 **4 5** +
TRAIL TYPE
Loop
SURFACE TYPE
Dirt

FEATURES
Dogs Allowed
Canyon
Mountain
Stream
Birds
Wildflowers
Wildlife
Great Views
Photo Opportunity
Historic
Geologic

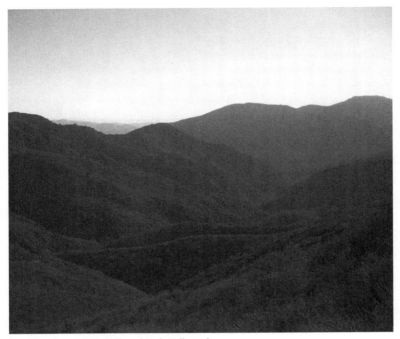

Looking down *to Big Falls and Little Falls creek canyons*

on West Pozo Road toward Santa Margarita when the highway branches off to the left. Follow West Pozo Road for another 2.0 miles, and look for the Rinconada Trail day-use parking area on the right.

Trail Description

 Horses

The trailhead is marked by a kiosk at the south end of the Rinconada Trail parking area. A **water trough and hitching post** have been placed near the trailhead for horses. ▶1

Follow the trail south, away from the mining area to the west, and stay on the main single track as it veers to the left at 0.23 mile. ▶2 Avoid the spur to the right, which heads down to the mine area.

The trail climbs 200 feet in the first 0.5 mile with a series of steep switchbacks that add to the challenge for riders on horseback or bike. The views down to Santa Margarita and Pozo improve with each switchback as you climb toward the origin of Little Falls Creek. The first mile of the trail is shaded by a mixed evergreen forest, which includes coast live and valley oak.

A trail marker signifies completion of the first mile, as the trail flattens out over the grassland portion of the hike, which is made more colorful in the spring when the **poppies** and **bush lupines** are in full bloom. Stay left as the marker suggests and continue to the summit. **Wildflowers**

You'll come to a cattle gate at 1.4 miles, ▶3 at an elevation of 2,360 feet. Make sure the gate closes on your way through. At this point, you've already climbed 567 feet. The trail follows the ridgeline at 1.5 miles, ▶4 looking down to **Big Falls and Little** **Canyon**

Rinconada Mine

NOTES

The U.S. Environmental Protection Agency closed the Rinconada Trail to the public on November 4, 2003, because of pollutants. The area was fenced off for a massive cleanup effort after soil samples at Rinconada Mine revealed high levels of mercury. The agency also made note of a handful of hazardous mining tunnels in the area. During the summer of 2005, the Rinconada Trail—which runs to the south, away from the mine—was reopened to the public with no potential health risks listed by the EPA. The mine area, however, was still closed at the time of this book's production.

The EPA encourages trail users to abide by the signs and fences posted in the Rinconada Mine area, avoiding the mine site, about 0.1 mile west of the trailhead.

The Rinconada Mine was opened in 1872 when cinnabar veins were discovered in the area. The Rinconada site was worked until the early 1960s, and some mining equipment can still be seen in the area.

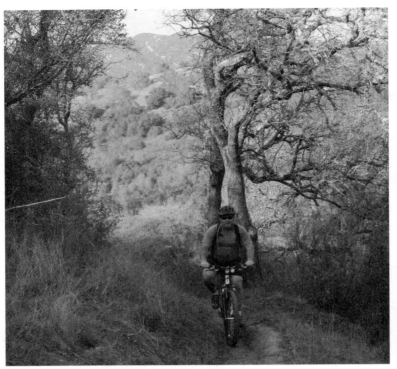

The Rinconada Trail *is a fun ride for mountain bikers.*

Falls canyons. The two creeks are feeder streams of Lopez Creek, the main supplier of water to Lopez Lake—located 3.5 miles to south. Remember this viewpoint, marked by a pile of rocks topped with a brown trail marker. The trail will loop back to this point in a clockwise fashion in 1.75 miles.

For now, continue straight ahead along on the ridgeline, following the main single track to a dirt road ▶5 at the 2.0-mile mark. Make a right on the access road and follow it downhill (southwest) toward Little Falls Canyon.

At 2.8 miles, the road passes over **Little Falls Creek**, which originates at a nearby spring about

 Stream

400 feet north of the creek crossing. The trail loops back to the ridgeline via a spur on the right side of the dirt road at 2.9 miles. ►6 The trail is clearly marked with another marker.

After 3.25 miles, the climb brings you to the main trail again, near the marker you took notice of at the 1.5-mile mark. This completes the mini-loop. ►7 Follow the single track north in the same fashion you came to return to the parking area. You'll know you're on the right track when you pass through the cattle gate again at 3.33 miles.

MILESTONES

►1	0.00	Follow the trail south, past hitching post and trough.
►2	0.23	Stay left and ignore spur to the mine area.
►3	1.40	Pass cattle gate, closing it behind you.
►4	1.50	Take note of trail marker and continue along ridge trail.
►5	2.00	Trail runs into a dirt road; follow it downhill toward Little Falls Creek.
►6	2.90	After the creek, a spur on the right-hand side climbs back to the ridge.
►7	3.25	Complete the loop and return the way you came from the north.

Hi Mountain

OPTIONS

A fire road located 2.0 miles into the Rinconada Trail can be taken to the east (uphill) for 4.0 miles to Hi Mountain, one of the highest summits in the area at, 3,199 feet. A condor lookout station has been built on this crest of the Santa Lucia Mountains. Call (805) 748-3199 for more information on the Hi Mountain Lookout.

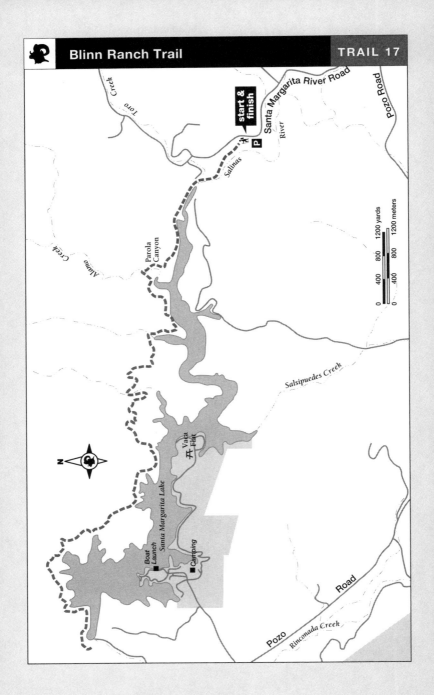

Blinn Ranch Trail

TRAIL 17

Toro Creek

Santa Margarita River Road

Pozo Road

start & finish

P

Salinas River

Parola Canyon

Alamo Creek

Salsipuedes Creek

N

Vaca Flat

Santa Margarita Lake

Boat Launch

Camping

Pozo Road

Rinconada Creek

0   400   800   1200 yards
0   400   800   1200 meters

Blinn Ranch Trail

One of longest multiuse trails on the Central Coast, the 18-mile Blinn Ranch Trails runs around the north side of Santa Margarita Lake and is popular with mountain bikers and horseback riders. The trail takes users to of a side of the lake that is rarely seen by the public, which usually sticks to the south shore.

Best Time

The trail is open during daylight hours all year, although it will be closed during and shortly after storms to protect it. Portions of the trail could get flooded by the Salinas River during the rainy season. The weather here gets hot in the summer, surpassing 100°F, and there is no swimming permitted at the lake, so bring plenty of water.

Finding the Trail

From Hwy. 101 in San Luis Obispo, head north over the Cuesta Grade and take the Santa Margarita exit, which becomes Hwy. 58. Take the highway through town for 1.6 miles, turning right over the railroad tracks, toward Santa Margarita Lake. Stay on the highway for another 1.6 miles, but then, when the highway branches off to the left, stay straight on West Pozo Road toward Santa Margarita. Follow West Pozo Road for another 9.0 miles past Santa Margarita Lake toward Pozo. Look for the RIVER ROAD ACCESS sign immediately after crossing the bridge over the Salinas River and make a left on Santa Margarita River Road. The day-use parking

TRAIL USE
Hike, Run, Bike, Horse
LENGTH
18 miles, all day
VERTICAL FEET
±600
DIFFICULTY
− 1 2 3 4 **5** +
TRAIL TYPE
Out & Back
SURFACE TYPE
Mixed

FEATURES
Dogs Allowed
Stream
Lake
Birds
Wildflowers
Wildlife
Great Views
Camping
Secluded
Parking Fee

FACILITIES
Restrooms
Picnic Tables
Campground

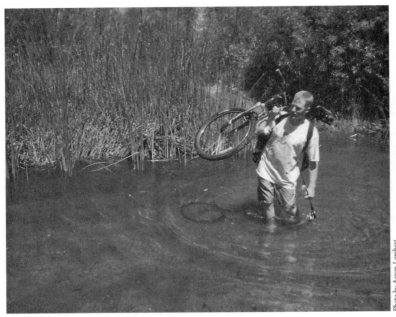

The Blinn Ranch Trail *includes a couple creek crossings.*

lot is on the left-hand side at 2.2 miles. There is a day-use fee.

Trail Description

🐎 **Horses**

The trailhead is at the **livestock gate** toward the tail end of the dirt parking lot. Be sure the gate is closed after you pass through. ►1 The trail starts as a fire road running alongside the Salinas River. Santa Margarita Lake was formed by the dam on the river, which can flood after a heavy storm.

The road, which is made up of washed-out pavement, gravel, and dirt, meets up with the Blinn Ranch Trail at 0.5 mile. ►2 Take a right and follow the single track toward the lake. The road continues left to the Sandstone Trail. The single track passes

the remains of an old ranch house at 0.7 mile and
crosses a wooden-deck footbridge over a **creek** at   Stream
0.8 mile. ▶3

Continue to the first visible finger of the lake
at 1.3 miles. ▶4 The trail follows the perimeter of
the lake and crosses Alamo Creek at 1.8 miles. ▶5
Continue around the lake until you come to a junction with the Cold Canyon Trail at 3.5 miles. Cold
Canyon Trail, which veers off to the left, heads down
to a hike-in campground near the water's edge. You
stay straight on the fire road. ▶6

At 4.8 miles, the trail passes another cattle gate
▶7 and continues on to the middle portion of the
lake, across from Vaca Flat. During the production   ≋ Lake
of this book, there was a new trail being constructed
at about the 6.0-mile mark, which will give access

Shorter, Multiuse Trails

OPTIONS

If the Blinn Ranch Trail is too much to handle, there is also a handful
of shorter, multiuse trails at Santa Margarita Lake.

Trails accessible via the River Road parking area include the
Sapwi/Cold Canyon and Sandstone trails.

- The 3.4-mile Sapwi Trail branches off of the Blinn Ranch Trail at
  the 3.5-mile mark and runs down to Khus and Sapwi camps.

- The 5.4-mile Sandstone Trail turns off the main fire road at the
  trailhead, near the parking area.

There are three trails accessible via the main entrance to the
lake, off Santa Margarita Lake Road.

- The Grey Pine Trail is 3.3 miles one way to Vaca Flat.

- The Lakeside Trail is an unmarked dirt road that circles counterclockwise from the marina around the point and back to the
  White Oak campground.

Another popular trail is Rocky's Trail, which starts near the main
entrance and heads 1.8 miles out toward the dam.

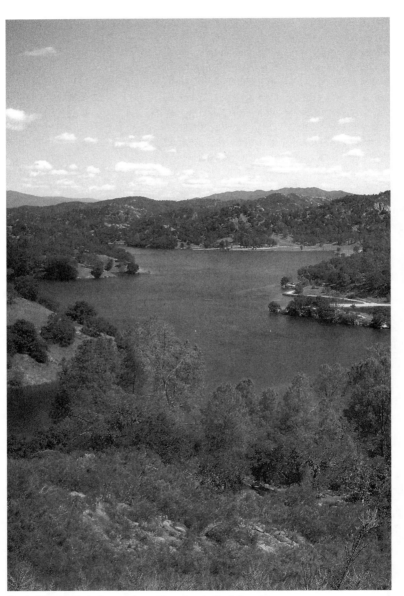

Santa Margarita Lake *was formed by a dam in the Salinas River.*

to a previously unreachable portion of the Santa Margarita backcountry.

The turnaround is at a gate that separates the trail from private property at 9.0 miles. ▶8 Follow the trail back to the parking area, which closes at dark.

Notice

Camping is available in the Coyote, Roadrunner, Grey Pine, and Osprey campgrounds at the south end of Santa Margarita Lake—accessible via Santa Margarita Lake Road. The Sapwi and Khus campgrounds on the north side of the lake are primitive sites that can be reserved ahead of time. Call (805) 788-2397 to make reservations.

🚶	MILESTONES	
▶1	0.0	The trailhead is at the livestock gate at the parking lot.
▶2	0.5	Make a right off the service road onto the Blinn Ranch Trail.
▶3	0.7	Cross the wooden-deck bridge and feeder creek.
▶4	1.3	Catch your first glimpse of the lake, continuing down the trail.
▶5	1.8	Cross Alamo Creek and cruise uphill toward Cold Canyon.
▶6	3.5	Stay straight at the intersection with Cold Canyon Trail.
▶7	4.8	Pass another cattle gate and continue around the perimeter of the lake.
▶8	9.0	The trail ends at a lake marking private property; this is the turnaround.

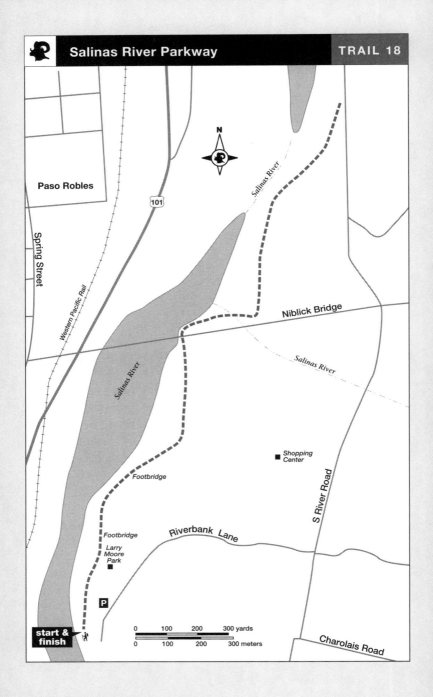

Salinas River Parkway — TRAIL 18

Paso Robles

101

Spring Street

Western Pacific Rail

Salinas River

Salinas River

Niblick Bridge

Salinas River

Footbridge

Shopping Center

S River Road

Footbridge

Riverbank Lane

Larry Moore Park

P

start & finish

| 0 | 100 | 200 | 300 yards |
| 0 | 100 | 200 | 300 meters |

Charolais Road

Salinas River Parkway

With all the residential and retail development taking place in the North County, city trails like the Salinas River Parkway in Paso Robles are becoming increasing precious. A silver lining of the Niblick Bridge Project and the Wal-Mart shopping center, this riverside trail was developed as part of a statewide project to improve California river parkways, funded by a resources bond known as the California Clean Water, Clean Air, Safe Neighborhood Parks, and Coastal Protection Act of 2002.

Best Time

Because it is one of the few public trails in Paso Robles, the parkway is well maintained throughout the year. Many local residents use the trail in the evening to walk their dogs after work. Morning hikes during the week are best for hikers searching for seclusion.

Finding the Trail

From San Luis Obispo, drive 28 miles north and take the Niblick Road exit. Take a right over the Niblick Bridge, crossing the Salinas River and driving past the Wal-Mart shopping center. After 0.6 mile, make another right on South River Road and follow it for 0.3 mile. Take a right on Riverbank Lane and follow it to the end of the cul-de-sac where the trailhead is located.

TRAIL USE
Hike, Run, Bike
LENGTH
2.2 miles, 1.0 hour
VERTICAL FEET
±80
DIFFICULTY
− 1 **2** 3 4 5 +
TRAIL TYPE
Out & Back
SURFACE TYPE
Mixed

FEATURES
Handicap Access
Child Friendly
Dogs Allowed
Stream
Fall Color
Birds
Wildflowers
Wildlife

Trail Description

The trail begins at the end of Riverbank Lane and weaves through grassy Larry Moore Park, ▶1 paralleling the river on the left-hand side as you head toward the Niblick Bridge. Going through the park, the path crosses **small footbridges** ▶2 at the 0.15-, 0.25- and 0.55-mile marks. A spur on the right after the third bridge heads up to the shopping center.

The trail leaves the park environment and takes you strolling alongside the riverbed to a paved bike path, which passes under the bridge at 0.6 mile. ▶3 After the bridge, the trail turns to dirt again and pulls away from the streambed area, climbing a couple of switchbacks and skipping past another retail development on the south end of Paso Robles.

The final leg of the trail wanders beneath shady oak groves and looks down to where the river should be. The Salinas usually does not flow above ground for more than a couple months of the year, as it is a largely underground water source. Follow the path downstream until it meets up with another **paved bike path** at 0.8 mile. ▶4 The trail rolls through another residential area and ends at a cul-de-sac just after the 1.0-mile mark, which is the turnaround. ▶5

 Child Friendly

The Salinas River Parkway is one of the first trails brought about by the Upper Salinas River Corridor Enhancement project.

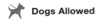 **Dogs Allowed**

★	MILESTONES	
▶1	0.00	Head north through Larry Moore Park.
▶2	0.15	Cross the first of three footbridges near the park.
▶3	0.60	The trail passes under Niblick Bridge.
▶4	0.80	Path continues north to a paved bike path.
▶5	1.10	A cul-de-sac marks the turnaround.

NOTES

The River

The Salinas River begins in the La Panza Range, located east of San Luis Obispo, continues down to the dam at Santa Margarita Lake and flows north through Atascadero and Paso Robles on its way up to Monterey. It is one of the few north-flowing rivers in the West.

Southern San Luis Obispo County

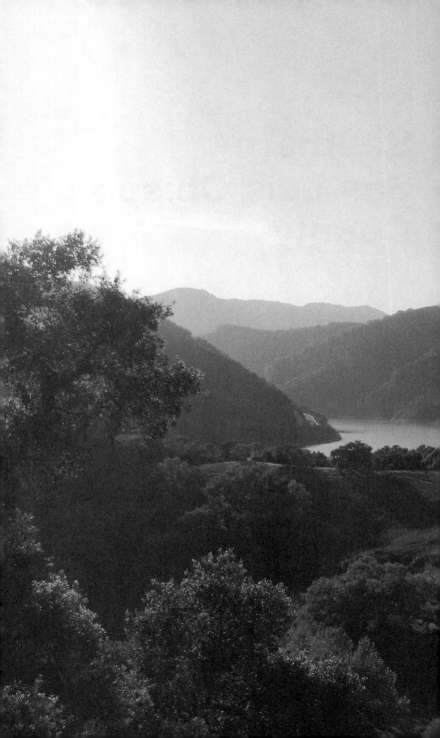

Southern San Luis Obispo County

The city of San Luis Obispo is located in the heart of the Central Coast. It offers dozens of dayhikes that many locals retreat to before work, after work, or on their lunch breaks, in some cases. Two of the Central Coast's signature hikes, Bishop Peak and Cerro San Luis, are located right in the middle of town and offer amazing, 360-degree views of the county. The two peaks are part of San Luis Obispo County's Nine Sisters, a set of volcanic plugs that run in a row from Morro Bay to San Luis Obispo. Next to Morro Rock, Bishop Peak and Cerro San Luis are the most recognizable peaks in the system.

Another popular San Luis Obispo landmark is Cuesta Grade, which has an elevation rise of more than 1,400 feet and is a popular climb and downhill ride for local cyclists. West Cuesta Ridge splits the northern and southern portions of the county and runs all the way to the Cerro Alto Campground between Morro Bay and Atascadero. The narrow access road atop the ridge is a favorite getaway for mountain bikers, providing spectacular views of the entire county.

The eastern portion of the ridgeline runs to Lopez Canyon, where two of the county's top backcountry hikes can be found. Turkey Ridge to Blackberry Springs is one of the many multiuse trails at Lopez Lake. Just north of the lake, the Big Falls Trail leads to an 80-foot waterfall in the isolated Santa Lucia Wilderness.

The last three hikes in this chapter are along the coast. The Oso Flaco Lake, Pismo Beach Monarch Grove, and Bob Jones City to Sea trails are relatively short, flat hikes that are great for the whole family.

Permits and Maps

Cuesta Ridge and its accompanying hikes are considered part of the Santa Lucia Ranger District of the Los Padres National Forest. A National Forest

Overleaf and opposite: *Looking down to Lopez Lake and the campground from Turkey Ridge*

Adventure Pass is required for some Los Padres hikes, although the program is being phased out in some areas. The pass can be purchased at ranger stations and area sporting goods retailers, including Big 5 in San Luis Obispo and Paso Robles. The $30 passes also can be ordered by calling (909) 382-2622.

Los Padres National Forest maps can be viewed at www.fs.fed.us/r5/forestvisitormaps/lospadres or purchased at www.nationalforeststore.com. For more information, contact the Los Padres ranger station in Goleta at (805) 968-6640.

The Eagle Rock Trail is in El Chorro Regional Park, where there is a day-use fee. Trail maps can be found at the entrance kiosk or near the signed trailhead. The Bishop Peak, Cerro San Luis and Bob Jones trails are city open-space projects. Maps are available at www.slocity.org. For more information, call the San Luis Obispo Parks and Recreation Department at (805) 781-7300.

There is a day-use fee for hikes within the Lopez Lake Recreation Area. A map and trail brochure can be picked up at ranger station located at the park entrance. The Pismo Beach Monarch Grove is run by the city. The grove is located right off Hwy. 1, and additional information is available at the visitors center.

Oso Flaco Lake is actually part of the Oceano Dunes State Vehicle Recreation Area, although the southern portion of the park is off-limits to off-road vehicles. There is a day-use fee to park in the lot near the trailhead, which is far removed from the off-road section to the north. A map and brochure are available at the entrance kiosk.

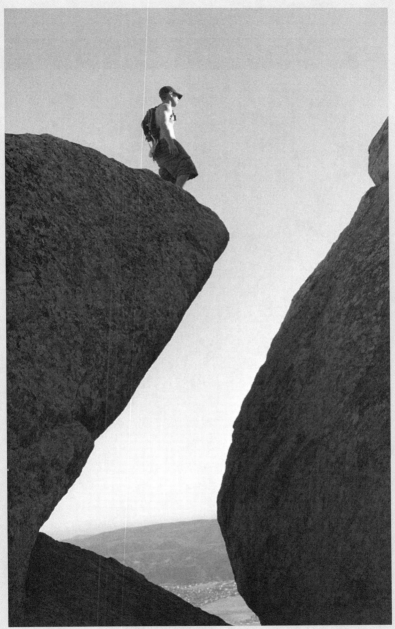

Bishop Peak *is a popular spot for rock climbing.*

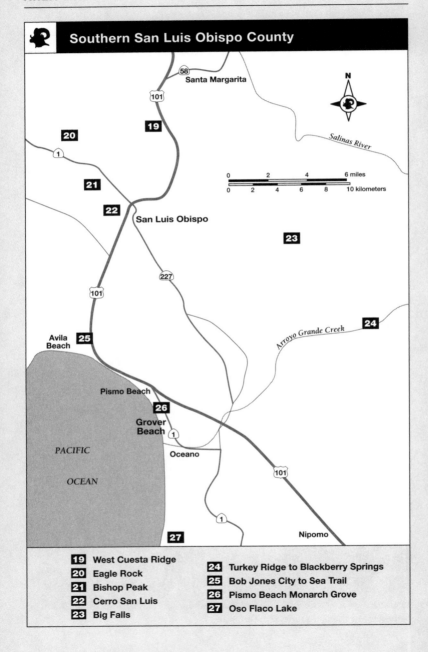

Southern San Luis Obispo County

19

20

1

21

22

San Luis Obispo

Santa Margarita

58

101

Salinas River

N

0   2   4   6 miles
0   2   4   6   8 10 kilometers

23

227

Avila
Beach

25

Pismo Beach

26

Grover
Beach

1

Oceano

Arroyo Grande Creek

24

101

PACIFIC

OCEAN

1

Nipomo

27

19 West Cuesta Ridge
20 Eagle Rock
21 Bishop Peak
22 Cerro San Luis
23 Big Falls

24 Turkey Ridge to Blackberry Springs
25 Bob Jones City to Sea Trail
26 Pismo Beach Monarch Grove
27 Oso Flaco Lake

TRAIL FEATURE TABLE

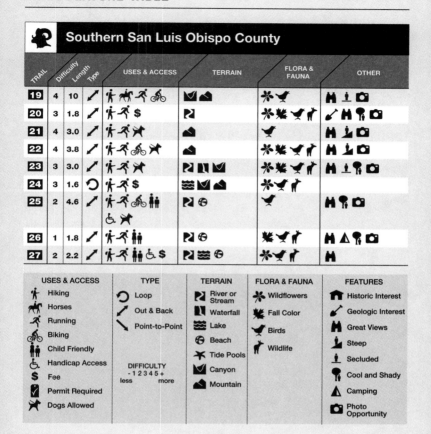

Southern San Luis Obispo County

TRAIL	Difficulty	Length	Type	USES & ACCESS	TERRAIN	FLORA & FAUNA	OTHER
19	4	10	↗	🚶 🐎 🏃 🚲	Canyon, Mountain	Wildflowers, Birds	Great Views, Steep, Photo
20	3	1.8	↗	🚶 🏃 $	River	Wildflowers, Fall Color, Birds, Wildlife	Geologic Interest, Great Views, Cool and Shady, Photo
21	4	3.0	↗	🚶 🏃 🐕	Mountain	Birds	Great Views, Steep, Photo
22	4	3.8	↗	🚶 🏃 🚲 🐕	Canyon	Wildflowers, Fall Color, Birds, Wildlife	Great Views, Steep, Photo
23	3	3.0	↗	🚶 🏃 🐕	River, Waterfall, Canyon	Wildflowers, Fall Color, Birds, Wildlife	Great Views, Secluded, Cool and Shady, Photo
24	3	1.6	↻	🚶 🏃 $	Lake, Canyon, Mountain	Wildflowers, Birds	
25	2	4.6	↗	🚶 🏃 🚲 👪 ♿ 🐕	River, Beach	Birds	Great Views, Cool and Shady, Photo
26	1	1.8	↗	🚶 🏃 👪	River, Beach	Fall Color, Wildlife	Great Views, Camping, Cool and Shady, Photo
27	2	2.2	↗	🚶 🏃 👪 ♿ $	River, Lake, Beach	Wildflowers, Wildlife	Great Views

USES & ACCESS	TYPE	TERRAIN	FLORA & FAUNA	FEATURES
🚶 Hiking	↻ Loop	River or Stream	Wildflowers	Historic Interest
🐎 Horses	↗ Out & Back	Waterfall	Fall Color	Geologic Interest
🏃 Running	↘ Point-to-Point	Lake	Birds	Great Views
🚲 Biking		Beach	Wildlife	Steep
👪 Child Friendly		Tide Pools		Secluded
♿ Handicap Access	DIFFICULTY	Canyon		Cool and Shady
$ Fee	- 1 2 3 4 5 +	Mountain		Camping
Permit Required	less more			Photo Opportunity
🐕 Dogs Allowed				

Southern San Luis Obispo County

TRAIL 19

Hike, Run, Bike, Horse
10 miles, 5.0 hours
Out & Back
Difficulty: 1 2 3 **4** 5

A popular ride for mountain bikers, West Cuesta Ridge divides northern and southern San Luis Obispo County, running from Cuesta Pass to Cerro Alto. The Los Padres National Forest trail follows partially paved TV Tower Road and tops out at the 2,600-foot mark, winding through a botanical garden and offering outstanding views of both sides of the county.

TRAIL 20

Hike, Run
1.8 miles, 1.0 hour
Out & Back
Difficulty: 1 2 **3** 4 5

Eagle Rock can be seen from Hwy. 1, protruding from the hillside high above El Chorro Regional Park. The trail to the rock, which might be better named Hawk Rock because of all the red-tailed hawks in the area, is a popular workout for nearby students at Cuesta College and for National Guard members at Camp San Luis Obispo.

TRAIL 21

Hike, Run
3.0 miles, 1.5 hours
Out & Back
Difficulty: 1 **2** 3 4 5

This is one of two signature hikes in San Luis Obispo. Certainly one of the most recognizable peaks in the region, Bishop Peak earned its name from the three points at the summit, which resemble a bishop's miter. One of the most popular of the Nine Sisters, Bishop is a favorite with rock climbers, hikers, and runners.

Cerro San Luis 159

The other signature San Luis Obispo is Cerro San Luis, a 1,292-foot morro also known as Madonna Mountain and San Luis Mountain. The old access road to the summit winds around the mountain and offers expansive views of the city and nearby Bishop Peak, another other San Luis Obispo must-do-hike.

TRAIL 22

Hike, Run, Bike
3.8 miles, 2.0 hours
Out & Back
Difficulty: 1 2 3 **4** 5

Big Falls 165

A remote backcountry single track tucked between Lopez and Santa Margarita lakes, the Big Falls Trail follows the creek upstream to not one but two magnificent waterfalls. Getting to the trailhead, however, might be the biggest challenge, as there are a dozen creek crossings along Upper Lopez Canyon Road. Driving a small car is not advised when creek flows are up.

TRAIL 23

Hike, Run
3.0 miles, 1.5 hours
Out & Back
Difficulty: 1 2 **3** 4 5

Turkey Ridge to Blackberry Springs 169

This hike combines two of the best and most solitary trails about Lopez Lake, offering a panoramic view of the lake and the campsites sprinkled around its edges. Starting near the entrance to the lake, the multiuse trail crawls up the ridgeline before descending through the shaded Blackberry Spring Trail to the lower campground.

TRAIL 24

Hike, Run
1.6 miles, 1.0 hour
Loop
Difficulty: 1 2 **3** 4 5

Bob Jones City to Sea Trail 175

The City to Sea Trail is just that, a simple bike path that follows San Luis Obispo Creek to Port San Luis in Avila Beach. The two-lane paved path runs alongside the creek and golf course, spans a bridge over the widest part of the creek, and spits out near the white-sand beach day-use area.

TRAIL 25

Hike, Run, Bike
4.6 miles, 2.0 hours
Out & Back
Difficulty: 1 **2** 3 4 5

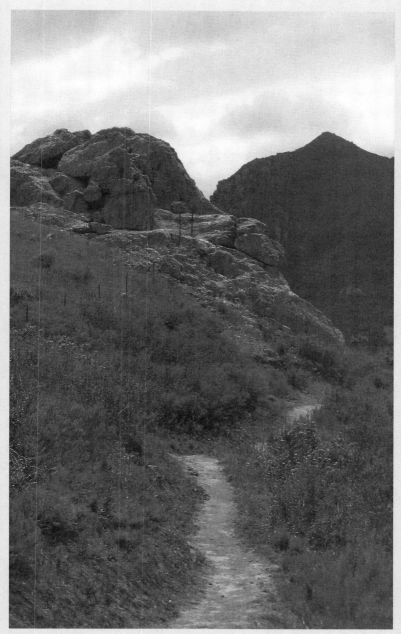

Eagle Rock *with Cerro Romauldo in the background*

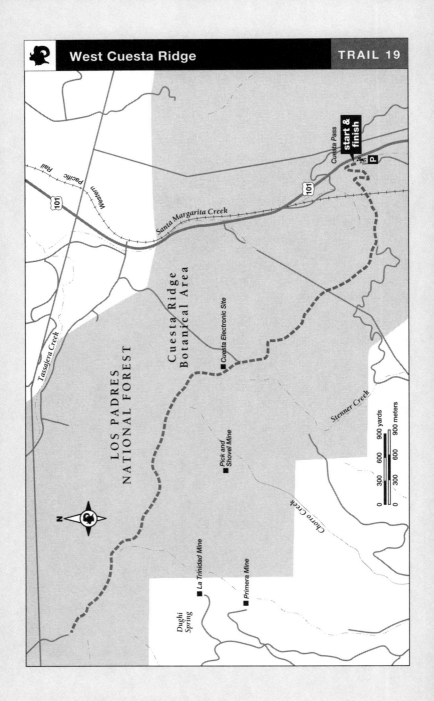

Cuesta Pass

start & finish

P

Cuesta Ridge Botanical Area

Cuesta Electronic Site

Santa Margarita Creek

Western Pacific Rail

Tassajera Creek

LOS PADRES NATIONAL FOREST

Pick and Shovel Mine

Stenner Creek

Chorro Creek

La Trinidad Mine

Primera Mine

Dughi Spring

N

0 300 600 900 yards
0 300 600 900 meters

West Cuesta Ridge

The West Cuesta Ridge Trail is the great divide between northern and southern San Luis Obispo County, running across the ridgetop from Cuesta Pass to Cerro Alto. This Los Padres National Forest trail crawls up above 2,500 feet and runs along partially paved TV Tower Road. A favorite of local mountain bikers because of the countless single tracks that branch off the main trail, the road also draws its share of botanists and sightseers, thanks to a 1,300-acre botanical area along with spectacular views of the golden coast and the chain of morros, which lead to the centerpiece of the county—San Luis Obispo.

Best Time

The ridge trail is ideal for sunrise and sunset rides and hikes, especially in the summer months when the heat keeps many trail users away. The botanical area is at its best in the late spring when the hills are green and the flowers are in full bloom.

Finding the Trail

Take Hwy. 101 north from San Luis Obispo to the dirt parking area at the summit of Cuesta Grade on the west side of the freeway. Park in the day-use area. The trail runs up TV Tower Road—also called West Cuesta Ridge Road.

TRAIL USE
Hike, Run, Bike, Horse
LENGTH
10 miles, 5.0 hours
VERTICAL FEET
±1010
DIFFICULTY
- 1 2 3 **4** 5 +
TRAIL TYPE
Out & Back
SURFACE TYPE
Dirt, Paved

FEATURES
Canyon
Mountain
Birds
Wildflowers
Great Views
Photo Opportunity
Secluded

Trail Description

Head north on TV Tower Road, ▶1 which starts at just over 1,500 feet and climbs another thousand feet by the time you reach the botanical area. At 0.5 mile, you'll pass a gate to a private residence. Stay to the left and continue the climb to the top of the ridge. At 1.25 miles, you'll pass a gate ▶2 and a dirt road that leads to a very technical **mountain biking trail** nicknamed "Shooters." Stay right and continue on up the paved road.

The climb continues with glimpses down to Poly Canyon, a popular destination for hiking/cycling college students at nearby Cal Poly. At 2.5 miles, the road passes another gate. This road leads to the television and radio antenna towers ▶3 that can be seen atop the ridge. Stay left on the paved road. The botanical area is right around the bend, at 2.8 miles.

 Biking

About a mile into the hike, views open up over Atascadero to the north and San Luis Obispo to the south.

 1994 Wildfire

NOTES

West Cuesta Ridge was hit hard by the Hwy. 41 wildfire in August 1994, which burned thousands of acres in the Los Padres National Forest. Unique plant species such as the Cuesta Pass Checkerbloom—a perennial herb with pinkish-lavender flowers that grows on serpentine rock and soils—are making a steady comeback, thanks to habitat conservation and other measures.

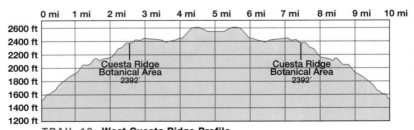

TRAIL 19   West Cuesta Ridge Profile

The Cuesta Ridge Botanical Area ▶4 was established in the late 1960s and contains about 1,334 acres of sensitive plant species that have been threatened by everything from wildfires to recreation and even mining practices. The signature plants among the coastal chaparral are the rare Sargent cypress and Cuesta Pass checkerbloom. The trail leaves the designated botanical area at the 5.0-mile mark, which is a good place to picnic and **look out over** Great Views **San Luis Obispo and the North Coast**. The road is pretty beat up after this point, which makes it a good turnaround spot. Follow the same road back to the parking area. ▶5

🚶	**MILESTONES**	
▶1	0.0	Begin your climb up TV Tower Road, initially traveling north.
▶2	1.3	Stay right when you reach the gated dirt road to "Shooters."
▶3	2.5	Continue down the paved road past the television and radio towers.
▶4	2.8	Enter the Cuesta Ridge Botanical Area.
▶5	5.0	Exit the botanical area, turn around, and return by the same route.

East Cuesta Ridge

The East Cuesta Ridge Trail is similar to the west-ridge version, minus the botanical garden and the full views of the North Coast. The trailhead is across Hwy. 101 from the West Cuesta Ridge Trail at East Cuesta Ridge Road, which is also known as Mount Lowe Road. Park just past the summit of Cuesta Grade at the turnout, to the right of the northbound lane. Don't block the gate.

The trail starts at the gate and continues on an easy-to-follow fire road toward Lopez Canyon. The unpaved road climbs up the ridge through a terrain that's similar to the West Ridge but sees less traffic. The road continues for about 7.0 miles before ending at private property.

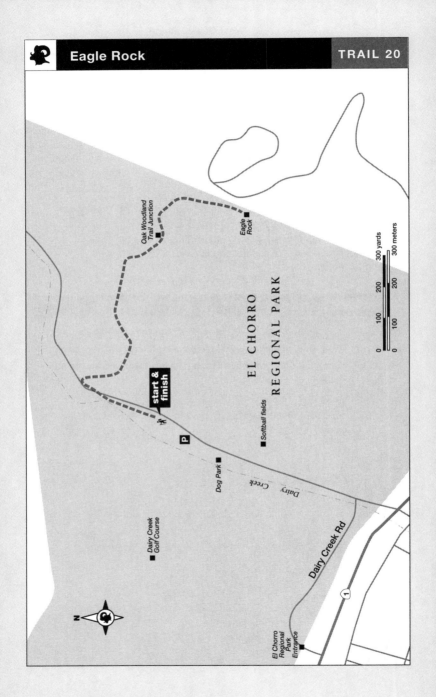

Oak Woodland
Trail Junction

Eagle
Rock

EL CHORRO

REGIONAL PARK

300 yards

0   100   200   300 meters

0   100   200

start &
finish

P

Softball fields

Dog Park

Dairy Creek

Dairy Creek

Dairy Creek
Golf Course

Dairy Creek Rd

1

El Chorro Regional
Park Entrance

N

Eagle Rock

The hike, or in this case sprint, to Eagle Rock used to be the punishment Cougars coaches handed out when they heard athletes were missing classes or failing exams at nearby Cuesta Community College in San Luis Obispo. It's been known as a popular conditioning run for members of the California National Guard at nearby Camp San Luis Obispo as well. Today, the trail is routed through the riparian habitat along Dairy Creek. Running through the coast live oaks and seasonal wildflowers, the self-guided nature trail to Eagle Rock offers precious panoramic views of the golf course, college, and military base nearby.

Best Time

This is a fun, year-round hike. Bring water on hot afternoons.

Finding the Trail

From Hwy. 101 in San Luis Obispo, take the Hwy. 1 exit and head north on Hwy. 1. Take the highway 5.5 miles past Cal Poly and the men's colony to the signed entrance to El Chorro Regional Park, on the east side of the highway, opposite Cuesta College. Make a right onto Dairy Creek Road and stay right to the park's entrance, avoiding the road to Dairy Creek Golf Course. There is a day-use fee at the park entrance on weekends and holidays during the main season. Continue past the entrance, the fields, and a dog park to the dirt parking area near the trailhead at the end of the drive. Pick up a map and nature

TRAIL USE
Hike, Run

LENGTH
1.8 miles, 1.0 hour

VERTICAL FEET
±425

DIFFICULTY
− 1 2 **3** 4 5 +

TRAIL TYPE
Out & Back

SURFACE TYPE
Dirt

FEATURES
Parking Fee
Stream
Fall Color
Birds
Wildflowers
Wildlife
Cool & Shady
Great Views
Photo Opportunity
Geologic

FACILITIES
Restrooms
Picnic Tables
Water
Phone
Campground

trail brochures at the kiosk to the left of the gated trail entrance.

Trail Description

After picking up a nature trail brochure, pass through the gate and follow the access road that parallels **Dairy Creek** to the east. ▶1 Follow the dirt road for about 0.15 mile to a single-track turnoff to Eagle Rock. ▶2 The trailhead, which is on the right-hand side, is clearly marked. From here, the trail climbs to the southeast, toward a canopy of oaks. A wooden handrail and some stone steps have been placed at the 0.3-mile mark, where hikers can look out to the golf course across Dairy Creek and Camp San Luis Obispo, Cerro Romauldo, and Cuesta College across Hwy. 1.

The trail levels out for a bit just before the 0.5-mile mark, ▶3 where you can look up to Eagle Rock to the south. The trail passes a spur to the Oak Woodland Trail at 0.52 mile. Stay right and continue the **climb up to the rock**. The trail legally passes through a fence and cattle guard at 0.7 mile, ▶4 where you can look north to Morro Rock and the three 450-foot smokestacks that tower above the Duke Energy power plant.

Eagle Rock is less than 0.25 mile away. Stay straight on the main trail and ignore the trail spur off to the left near the end of the trail. This spur leads to an overgrown single track that passes onto military property. At 0.9 mile, you'll reach the rock. A bench was placed at the base of the rock in April 2007 for hikers who could use a break or who just want to gaze out over Hwy. 1 as it weaves past the morros on its way to the North Coast. The elevation at the base of the large, reddish-brown, triangular rock is 725 feet. Avoid scaling the rock, which is a tempting climb but also is set on military land. Return the way you came. ▶5

Stream

Great Views

Eagle Rock is a popular training trail for local college athletes and the National Guard.

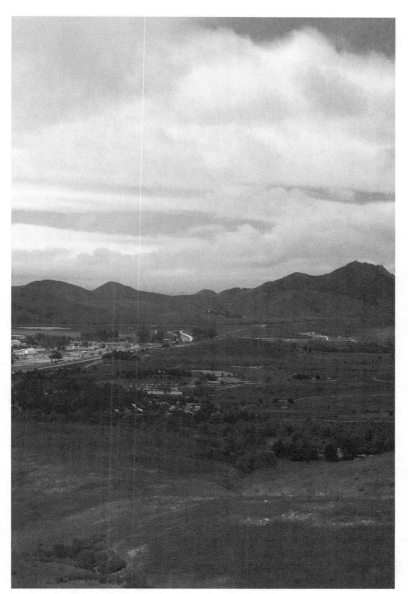

The bench at Eagle Rock *looks down to northern San Luis Obispo.*

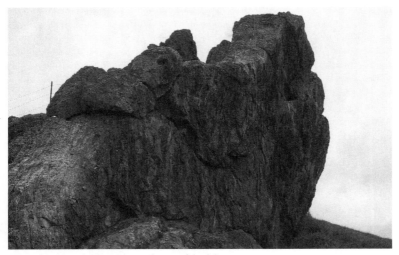

Eagle Rock *marks the turnaround point of this hike.*

Notice

El Chorro Regional Park offers a day-use area with barbecue facilities, volleyball courts, horseshoe pits, a dog park, botanical garden, and softball fields. Eagle Rock gets its name from the nearby outline of a giant eagle on the hillside just north of the red rock outcroppings at the trail's turnaround. The rocks, which are red, white, and blue, are arranged to form the shape of an eagle. This landmark, which is not visible from the trail, can best be seen from Hwy. 1.

🚶	**MILESTONES**	
►1	0.0	Pick up a trail brochure and follow the fire road east.
►2	1.5	The Eagle Rock Trailhead is on the right.
►3	0.5	Trail flattens out and passes the Oak Woodland Trailhead.
►4	0.7	Pass through a gate in the fence and continue up to Eagle Rock.
►5	0.9	The red rock marks the end of the out-and-back hike.

OPTIONS

El Chorro Regional Park

This park has a couple of additional maintained trails on the east side of Hwy. 1. The trails pass through the local ranchlands, which were once dotted with grazing cattle. Camp San Luis Obispo trained in this area during World War II and the Korean Conflict, before the land was deeded to the county in 1972 as part of President Richard Nixon's "Legacy of Parks."

All of El Chorro's trails are moderate hikes that are less than 2.0 miles long. The Oak Woodland Trail is a 1.5-mile single track that is open to hiking only and accessible via the Eagle Rock Trail. The Dairy Creek Trail, off the initial fire road, is a 1.2-mile trail open to hikers and mountain bikers. The park also is home to the San Luis Obispo Botanical Garden. Call (805) 546-3501 for more information on personal tours of the main garden. The El Chorro Regional Park Campground has more than 60 campsites, including 44 with full hookups. The sites are available on a first-come, first-served basis; reservations may be made for larger groups. Call (805) 781-5930 for more information.

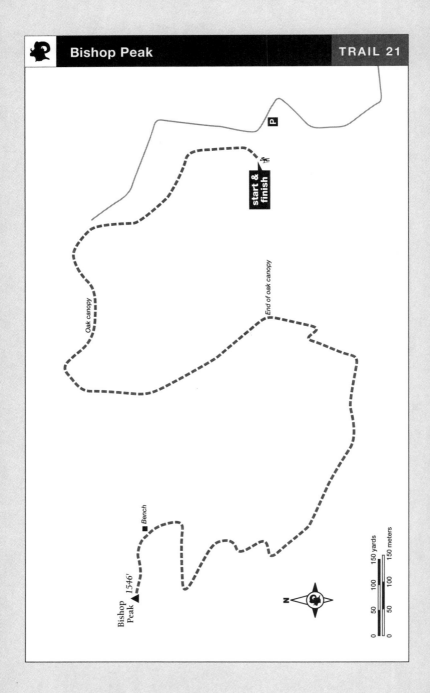

start & finish

P

Oak canopy

End of oak canopy

Bench

Bishop Peak ▲ 1546'

N

0   50   100   150 yards
0   50   100   150 meters

Bishop Peak

Bishop Peak and neighboring Cerro San Luis are San Luis Obispo's two signature hikes, offering amazing views of the city of San Luis Obispo and west, all the way to the Pacific. The peak is one of San Luis Obispo County's famed Nine Sisters, named in the late 18th century by the padres at Mission San Luis Obispo because of the three points on the summit, which resembles a bishop's miter.

Best Time

Because San Luis Obispo's weather is mild through-out the year, the trail is in good condition all year. Avoid hiking on rainy or extremely windy days. If afternoon wind gusts are whipping through the area, avoid rock hopping and climbing. Because the peak is located above 1,400 feet, with very few trees on the upper stretches, afternoon hikes can get rather warm.

Finding the Trail

From Hwy. 101 in San Luis Obispo, take the Santa Rosa St. exit and make a right on Santa Rosa. Make a left on Highland Dr., near Cal Poly, and follow it for another 4.0 miles until it ends at the Ferrini Ranch Open Space Trailhead. There are a couple other trailheads around the base of the hill. A popular access point off of Foothill Blvd., however, crosses private property, and that path is not maintained by the city.

TRAIL USE
Hike, Run
LENGTH
3.0 miles, 1.5 hours
VERTICAL FEET
±848
DIFFICULTY
– 1 2 3 **4** 5 +
TRAIL TYPE
Out & Back
SURFACE TYPE
Dirt

FEATURES
Dogs Allowed
Mountain
Steep
Birds
Great Views
Photo Opportunity

Trail Description

The beginning of the trail winds around a couple fences separating it from private residences before the trail meanders through the shade trees and rock formations that comprise the lower portions of the trail. ▶1 The rocks probably started up near the summit but tumbled down over time. Other boulders below were excavation casualties in the early 1900s, when the plug was mined heavily for its building stone.

Weave your way through the rocks and trees along the lower section of the preserve and stay left at the fork, at 0.15 mile, and follow the signed Bishop Peak Trail. ▶2 As you begin your climb, you can see the Cal Poly campus over your right shoulder, including Baggett Stadium, where the Cal Poly baseball team plays its home games in the spring.

Hang another left at 0.38 mile ▶3 and follow the single track that begins to wrap around the morro in a clockwise fashion. By 0.4 mile you're back under the oak canopy. That shade is long gone by 0.6 mile, where you emerge from the canopy and can see the city of San Luis Obispo below, along with neighboring Cerro San Luis across Foothill Blvd. ▶4 This is where the trail **really starts to climb**. At the 1.0-mile mark, Laguna Lake can be spotted in the distance. At 1.25 miles, you can see all the way

 Steep

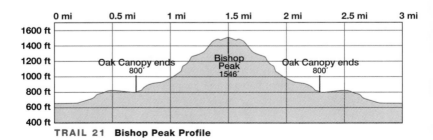

TRAIL 21 Bishop Peak Profile

down to the **South County** and spot the **Pacific Ocean** for the first time. ▶5

Great Views

After a half dozen switchbacks, you've just about reached the peak. A bench recognizing Jeff Bruckner, a climber who died here in April 2003, can be found at 1.5 miles. ▶6 You can reach the summit by doing some rock hopping, which will put you at an elevation of 1,546 feet. Return the way you came.

Notice

There are actually more than 20 peaks in the morros chain, a series of volcanic plugs that were formed some 20 million to 25 million years ago. Many local organizations, including the Santa Lucia Chapter of the Sierra Club, recognize just the nine major peaks. Those Nine Sisters are Morro Rock, Black Hill, Cabrillo Peak, Hollister Peak, Cerro Romauldo, Chumash Peak, Bishop Peak, Cerro San Luis, and Islay Hill.

🚶	MILESTONES	
▶1	0.00	Trail starts alongside fencing separating the single track from private property, then weaves through the oak canopy below.
▶2	0.15	Follow the signed Bishop Peak Trail by staying to your left.
▶3	0.38	Make another left and follow the narrow dirt trail clockwise back into the oak canopy.
▶4	0.60	The trail leaves the shady canopy and overlooks the city and Cerro San Luis.
▶5	1.25	The climb continues with a handful of steep switchbacks.
▶6	1.50	The summit is at 1,546 feet; it marks the end of the trail and the turnaround point.

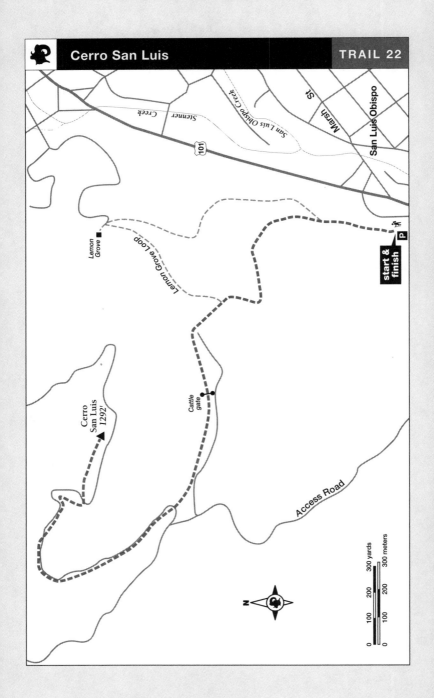

Cerro San Luis   **TRAIL 22**

San Luis Obispo

Marsh St

San Luis Obispo Creek

Stenner Creek

101

Lemon Grove

Lemon Grove Loop

start & finish

Cerro San Luis 1292'

Cattle gate

Access Road

N

0   100   200   300 yards
0   100   200   300 meters

Cerro San Luis

Also known as Madonna Mountain and as San Luis Mountain, this 1,292-foot morro is at the heart of San Luis Obispo and is one of the city's two signature hikes. The other hike, Bishop Peak, is across the street and can be seen as you wind your way up to the peak.

The mountain is set in the 118-acre Cerro San Luis Natural Reserve, with a trail that wraps around the entire perimeter of the mountain and offers 360-degree views of the city. It takes hikers and mountain bikers through several types of habitat—including grassland, coastal scrub, and oak woodland.

Best Time

This is a good year-round hike because much of it follows a well-maintained single track and a dirt access road. The wildflowers on the lower stretches of the hike are in full bloom during the spring. The mountain usually dries out by June and can be a sizzling trek during summer afternoons. Many locals hike the mountain during the holidays, particularly around Christmas and for a sunrise service on Easter Sunday.

Finding the Trail

From San Luis Obispo, Cerro San Luis is clearly marked by the large white "M" on the mountainside facing the Hwy. 101 freeway. The trailhead parking lot is just south of the Madonna Inn, at the west end of Marsh St. The easiest way to locate the parking lot is to take Hwy. 101 from northern San Luis Obispo

TRAIL USE
Hike, Run, Bike
LENGTH
3.8 miles, 2.0 hours
VERTICAL FEET
±1081
DIFFICULTY
– 1 2 3 **4 5** +
TRAIL TYPE
Out & Back
SURFACE TYPE
Dirt

FEATURES
Dogs Allowed
Mountain
Steep
Fall Color
Birds
Wildflowers
Wildlife
Great Views
Photo Opportunity

near Cal Poly to the Marsh St. exit. Immediately after exiting the freeway, take a left onto Fernandez Lane; then make an immediate right on Fernandez Road, which is really the parking area for the Cerro San Luis Trail. The trailhead is at the north end of the parking lot, past the gate.

Trail Description

The trail starts up the dirt access road and passes a spur to the Lemon Grove Loop at the onset. Stay straight on the main path and head north up to the summit, ▶1 leaving Hwy. 101 and the rest of the noise of the downtown area in your rearview. Keep a lookout for **mountain bikers**, especially on the single-track portion of the trail. The trail passes a cluster of prickly pear cactus and climbs to a bench at 0.25 mile. The bench is a nice point to pause at and take in the views of San Luis Obispo's downtown area.

Biking

At 0.35 mile, the trail makes a sharp turn to the right and continues to climb, and the views of the city improve with every step. At 0.5 mile, you pass another spur to the Lemon Grove Loop; this junction, at 452 feet, is the highest point of the loop. ▶2 Again, continue on the main single track toward the hilltop, staying left when the trail splits and heading west to a shady grove of oaks, which offers reprieve from the sun.

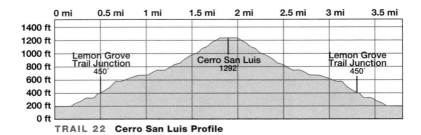

TRAIL 22   Cerro San Luis Profile

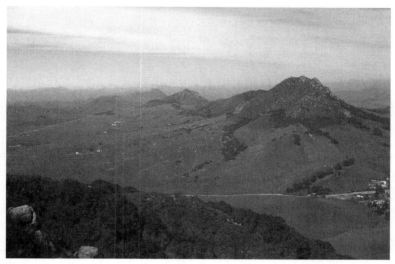

Bishop Peak, *located across Foothill Blvd., is the other signature hike in San Luis Obispo.*

After passing cattle gates at 0.6 and 0.75 mile, ►3 the single track finally starts feeling like a trail again, weaving through coastal scrub and winding around the west side of the mountain, far from the Alex Madonna Memorial Hwy. below. The large body of muddied water on the west side of town is Laguna Lake. A fire road descending to the lake peels off the main trail near the 1.0-mile mark. ►4 Stay right and continue the **climb to the top**. At 1.2 miles, you're at an elevation of 800 feet, which is just about eye level with the turkey vultures and other predatory birds that circle the mountaintop.

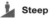 **Steep**

At 1.36 miles, the panoramic view stretches from Laguna Lake in the west to Bishop Peak to the north; the peak is another of the nine morros, which appear strategically stacked like pieces on a chessboard.

The trail splits again at 1.45 mile. ►5 Although each branch of the fork leads to the top, it's best to stay to the left and continue up the mountain

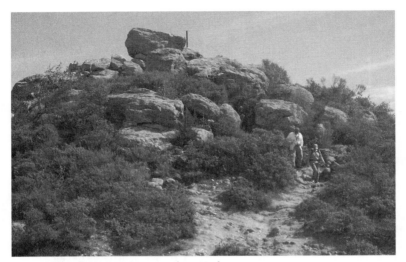

The peak can be reached *at just under 1,300 feet.*

in a clockwise fashion to get a roundabout view of the entire city. The Poly "P," located on the hillside behind Cal Poly to the east, shows you just how far you've come. The big letter can also be seen from the trailhead, which shows that the trail to the top has come full circle.

NOTES

Madonna Mountain

Cerro San Luis is often called Madonna Mountain in honor Alex Madonna, who owned the land the mountain sits on along with nearby Madonna Inn, a posh hotel that is a landmark of sorts for the city. Madonna died in 2004.

The White "M"

The white "M" on the hillside facing downtown is considered a historical landmark. Located in the Lemon Grove Open Space, the concrete "M" was built by Mission High students in 1965 and stands for the school and not, as many believe, Madonna Mountain.

The path tops out at 1.9 miles. Intermediate-level climbers can scale a few simple boulders to the summit, where an illuminated Christmas tree outline is anchored every winter. This is the end of the road. Return the way you came, ▶6 descending carefully down the mountain in a counterclockwise direction to the parking area.

⚶ MILESTONES

▶1   0.00   Pass the Lemon Grove Loop junction and continue climb to summit.

▶2   0.50   Pass another trail spur to the Lemon Grove and stay to the left at the fork.

▶3   0.60   The trail passes two gates.

▶4   1.00   Stay right, ignoring fire road down to the lake.

▶5   1.45   When the trail breaks, stick to the left fork to loop around to the summit.

▶6   1.90   After reaching the summit, retrace your steps to the parking area.

Lemon Grove Trail

OPTIONS

The Lemon Grove Loop is accessible via two spurs off the main summit trail on the eastern side of San Luis Mountain. The loop adds another mile to the summit trail. Most hikers take the main summit trail for 0.5 mile to the upper trailhead of the Lemon Grove trail because the loop is nearly all downhill from here.

The upper stretches of the loop pass a handful of lemon trees, for which the trail gets its name. The trail also has a couple batches of prickly pear cactus, a desert species producing colorful red blossoms that later ripen into fruit that is considered a delicacy by some Native Americans. Be sure to step aside when studying plants or watching wildlife, as this single track is a technical but popular downhill run for mountain bikers.

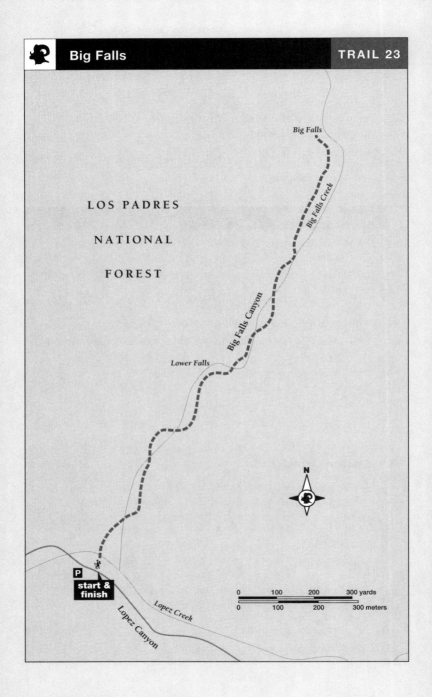

Big Falls

LOS PADRES

NATIONAL

FOREST

Big Falls Creek

Big Falls Canyon

Lower Falls

N

P
start & finish

Lopez Creek

Lopez Canyon

| 0 | 100 | 200 | 300 yards |
| 0 | 100 | 200 | 300 meters |

Big Falls

A pair of stunning waterfalls await those willing to make the trek to Big Falls Canyon and its gin-clear creek. Just driving to the trailhead at the confluence of Big Falls and Lopez creeks requires a dozen creek crossings along Upper Lopez Canyon Road. There are a couple more creek crossings waiting for you on the trail, but once you reach the first of the two waterfalls, the long drive is well worth the mud bath—just be sure to save time for a car wash afterward.

TRAIL USE
Hike, Run

LENGTH
3.0 miles, 1.5 hours

VERTICAL FEET
±340

DIFFICULTY
– 1 2 **3** 4 5 +

TRAIL TYPE
Out & Back

SURFACE TYPE
Dirt

Best Time

The waterfalls are most impressive in the spring, before stream flow drops in June and July. A shaded pool at the base of the lower falls is a nice resting spot in the summer, when inland temperatures can push 90°F.

FEATURES
Dogs Allowed
Canyon
Stream
Waterfall
Fall Color
Birds
Wildflowers
Wildlife
Cool & Shady
Great Views
Photo Opportunity
Secluded

Finding the Trail

Another tricky trailhead to find, the Big Falls Trailhead isn't marked by a sign but is located at then end of Upper Lopez Canyon Road. Small cars are not recommended on this road, which crosses the creek a dozen times. To get there, follow U.S. Hwy. 101 to Arroyo Grande and take the Hwy. 227 exit toward Lopez Lake. Take the highway east through town and bear right on Lopez Dr. just after the school. Follow the two-lane road for 10.3 miles to Lopez Lake. Just before the exit to Lopez Lake, hang a right on Hi Mountain Road and drive 0.8 mile to Upper Lopez Canyon Road. Make a left on

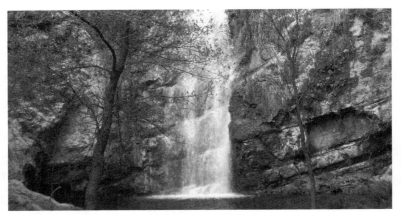

The lower falls *spills down the cliff along the Big Falls Trail.*

Upper Lopez Canyon Road and drive an adventurous 10 miles until the road dead-ends near the Big Falls trailhead. Park at the dirt turnout on the north side of the road near Lopez Creek.

Trail Description

From the parking area, follow the single track down to a crossing at Lopez Creek. ►1 The trail to the first waterfall follows **Big Falls Creek** to the north, weaving through a sycamore and oak forest. ►2 Along the way, the trail follows the creek upstream, passing numerous cascades and small pools that are home to tiny newts and wild rainbow trout.

To reach the smaller of the two falls, take a spur that goes left at the half-mile mark. ►3 The falls is quite impressive, at about 30 feet, with an enticing pool at a shady grove below.

While this waterfall is quite fulfilling, hikers should return to the main trail and continue north to the fall for which **Big Falls Canyon** is named.

The trail leaves the forested canyon and begins to flatten out after the first mile. At the 1.0-mile mark, the path leaves the shade and follows a rocky

Stream

Canyon

path upstream. The track crosses the creek several times and then runs between the canyon wall and the creek at 1.3 miles. ►4 Remain on the west side of the creek over the next 0.25 mile, passing a handful of smaller cascades before another spur leads down to the large falls at 1.5 miles ►5.

The 80-foot-high **Big Falls** is the most impressive waterfall in southern San Luis Obispo County. This is the turnaround, although the trail does continue north to Hi-Mountain Road, a fire road that is popular with four-wheelers and horseback riders.

 Waterfall

Notice

After heavy rains, the road to Big Falls, along with the trail itself, can be washed out. Call (805) 925-9538 for trail conditions.

🚶	**MILESTONES**	
►1	0.0	From parking area, head down to Lopez Creek.
►2	0.2	Trail follows tributary north through the canyon.
►3	0.5	Spur off main trail leads to lower falls.
►4	1.3	Trail crosses creek multiple times, continuing north.
►5	1.5	Another spur leads to Big Falls, the turnaround spot.

Little Falls

Two miles east of the Big Falls Trailhead, on the north side of Lopez Canyon Road, is a turnout for the Little Falls Trail. Little Falls is another impressive cascade, this one on Little Falls Creek, another tributary of Lopez Creek. The 50-foot cascade can be reached in 0.5 mile, making for a 1.0-mile round trip. Like the Big Falls Trail, the Little Falls Trail continues north to Hi-Mountain Road, which can be reached in 2.5 miles, near the lower reaches of the Rinconada Trail (Trail 16).

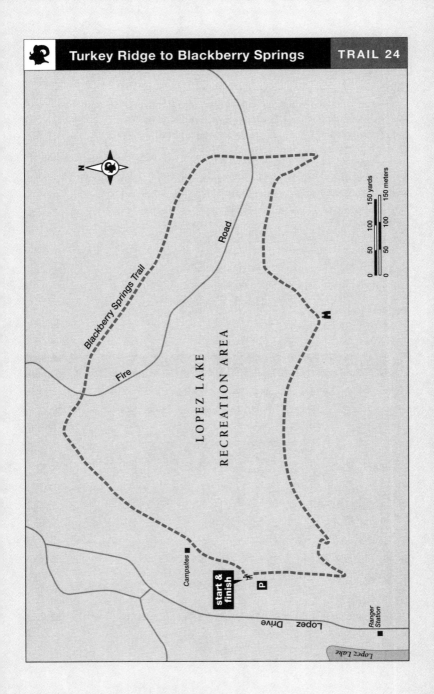

Turkey Ridge to Blackberry Springs **TRAIL 24**

N

Blackberry Springs Trail

Road

Fire

LOPEZ LAKE

RECREATION AREA

Campsites

start & finish

P

Lopez Drive

Ranger Station

Lopez Lake

0   50   100   150 yards
0   50   100   150 meters

Turkey Ridge to Blackberry Springs

This loop trail has a little bit of everything. It is a remote, quiet, single track that takes hikers far away from the pleasure boaters, campers, and waterslide fans nearby. The trail begins near the entrance to the Lopez Lake Recreation Area, climbing up to Turkey Ridge before it descends through the Blackberry Springs Trail to the lower campgrounds. The trails are fittingly named, as turkeys can often be seen and heard along the ridge route, and berries line the shady springs trail.

Best Time

The narrow trail can get overgrown with poison oak in the early spring. When hiking after the rainy season, check with the ranger staff to see if the single track has been maintained. Both trails are good year-round hikes. Keep in mind Lopez gets most of its activity in the summertime, when families flock to the lake and nearby waterslides to cool off.

Finding the Trail

From Hwy. 101 in Arroyo Grande, take the Grand Ave./Hwy. 227 exit and follow the highway through downtown Arroyo Grande for about 2.0 miles. Make a right at the stop sign and follow Lopez Dr. for 9.0 miles to the park entrance. The trailhead is on the far end of the parking lot, past the restrooms, near the main entrance. Park in the main parking lot and pay any day-use or parking fees at the walk-up window at the ranger station. Maps also are available at the ranger station.

TRAIL USE
Hike, Run

LENGTH
1.6 miles, 1.0 hour

VERTICAL FEET
±540

DIFFICULTY
– 1 2 **3** 4 5 +

TRAIL TYPE
Loop

SURFACE TYPE
Dirt

FEATURES
Parking Fee
Canyon
Mountain
Lake
Birds
Wildflowers
Wildlife

FACILITIES
Restrooms
Picnic Tables
Water
Phone
Campground

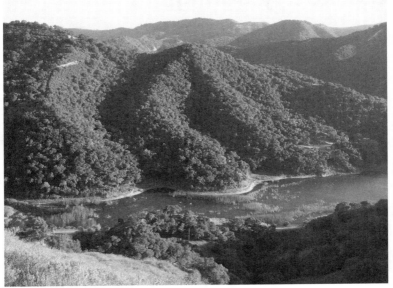

Turkey Ridge *sits high above the Arroyo Grande Arm of Lopez Lake.*

Trail Description

The trailhead is clearly marked at the north end of the lot, at an elevation of 520 feet. Follow the single track past the signed trailhead, ►1 climbing back south above the park entrance. At 0.1 mile, a clearing allows you to see all the way down to the lake and the campgrounds below. Be careful of poison oak on the lower sections of the trail and also throughout the Blackberry Springs portion, much of which runs through shaded groves and weaves through ferns and other berry bushes that are intertwined with poison oak.

The trail climbs 200 feet in the first 0.37 mile, ►2 entering an oak canopy that offers reprieve from the afternoon sun. The trail levels out a bit at the 0.5-mile mark (1060 feet) and is intersected by an

unmarked game trail. Follow the signed portion of
the trail by going straight. This portion of the trail
overlooks the Arroyo Grande Arm where Arroyo
Grande Creek dumps into the **lake**. The Arroyo **Lake**
Grande Arm and the creek area leading to it are
often closed to the public in the spring to protect the
spawning grounds of the largemouth bass. During
times when the area is roped off, you can only see it
from above, along Turkey Ridge.

The trail drops down to 932 feet at 0.67 mile
before shooting back up to the ridgeline. ▶3 A wall
of rock shale lines the left side of the trail at the
halfway mark. The trail descends to the Squirrel
and Eagle campgrounds from here. At 0.9 mile, turn

NOTES

Fishing at Lopez Lake

Lopez Lake can be one of the best fisheries San Luis Obispo County
has to offer. One deterrent, however, is the wind factor. Get out to
the lake early if you want to beat the breeze and take advantage of
this solid, year-round bass fishery. From late morning to late afternoon, frequent thermal winds can turn Lopez into a windsurfer's
paradise and an angler's worst nightmare.

The largemouth bite is typically rated "good" by the lake staff,
with crankbaits producing consistent results, while drop-shotting
plastic worms in the morning and chucking topwater lures in the
evening are productive options. The bigger fish are caught off rocky
points and deep creek drop-offs in the coves. Big bass also can be
caught down by the dam on Rat-L-Traps, MS Slammer lures, jerk
baits, and buzzbaits.

Shore anglers can catch smaller bass, which show near cover
and around brushy shoreline. Small crankbaits, Kastmasters, and
Rooster Tails fool shallow-water bass.

The lake also hosts the Lopez Lake Reel 'Em In Trout Derby and
receives trout plants throughout the winter and spring. Trout can be
caught on traditional spinners or PowerBait. When bass and trout
catches slow, many anglers focus on panfish, especially crappies,
which typically spawn later than bass.

onto the Blackberry Springs Trail, ▶4 which is the signed spur on the left, and drop down into a **shady tunnel** of oaks. At the 1.0-mile mark, you'll find a bench on your right.

There is one last climb, at 1.3 miles. ▶5 The trailhead to the Bobcat Trail is accessible via a spur on the right during this short climb. The trail you're on splits at 1.4 miles, although both forks meet up again shortly before the trail ends at 1.5 miles, at Lopez Dr. Follow the main road back to the main trailhead and parking lot, ▶6 which is at 1.6 miles.

Notice

There are more than 350 campsites at Lopez Lake, including primitive sites, those with electrical, and some offering full hook-ups. Reservations can be made up to one year in advance by calling (805) 788-2381.

MILESTONES

▶1	0.00	Trailhead is at the north end of the parking lot.
▶2	0.37	Trail climbs south, looking down at the main entrance and campgrounds.
▶3	0.67	After flattening out, the trail dips and climbs back to 932 feet at the halfway mark.
▶4	0.90	Follow the spur on the left to the Blackberry Springs Trail.
▶5	1.30	After one final climb, follow the trail down to Lopez Dr.
▶6	1.50	Follow the road through the campgrounds back to the parking lot.

Additional Lopez Lake Trails

There are at least seven additional maintained hiking trails within the Lopez Lake Recreation Area. A trail map is available at the ranger station.

- The Marina Trail, which is open to hikers and mountain bikers, is an easy 0.4-mile hike around the marina area.

- Rocky Point is another short, 0.4-mile trail that is open to hikers.

- Duna Vista (0.5 mile), Two Waters (1.3 miles), and Tuouski (1.8 miles) are other short hiking trails that offer outstanding views of the lake.

- High Ridge is one of the lake's most popular trails because it is open to horseback riding, mountain biking, and hiking. This 2.3-mile trail on the east side of the lake offers great views of the reservoir all the way down to the Arroyo Grande coast.

- Another favorite multiuse trail is the Wittenberg Arm Trail, a 1.0-mile climb into the Lopez backcountry that is popular with bird-watchers, geology enthusiasts, and mountain bikers.

A trailhead kiosk outlining the trail's route is located at the end of Lopez Dr. Two Waters, Duna Vista, and Tuouski trails are all accessible via the Wittenberg Arm Trail.

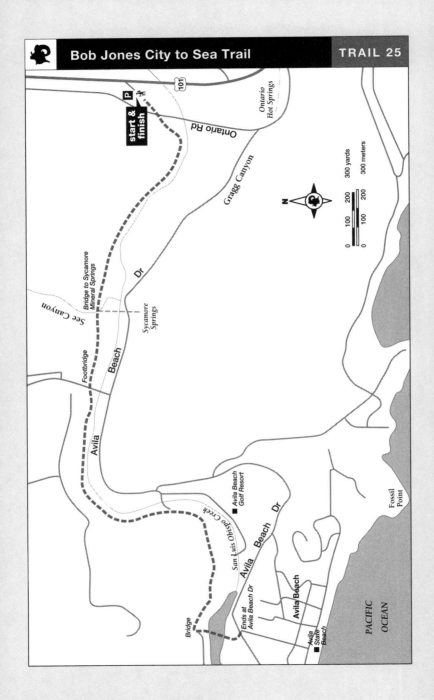

Bob Jones City to Sea Trail

TRAIL 25

Bob Jones City to Sea Trail

The Bob Jones City to Sea Trail is a popular bike path that runs from a parking lot near Hwy. 101 all the way to Avila Beach. The trail, appropriately named for a longtime Department of Fish and Game employee who fought to conserve the San Luis Obispo Creek habitat, parallels a creek that's home to such unique species as the southwest pond turtle, red-legged frog, and steelhead trout. The paved, two-lane path is used primarily by cyclists and walkers in the morning and evening hours.

Best Time

This path is open all year from sunrise to sunset and stays relatively cool throughout the year, particularly in the shady first half of the trail. Because the path is paved and well maintained, it's a good run or ride through all seasons.

Finding the Trail

From Hwy. 101 in San Luis Obispo, drive south to Avila Beach and exit at Avila Beach Dr. Make a right on Avila Beach Dr., heading toward the beach for 0.4 mile before making another right on Ontario Road. Follow the signs to the Bob Jones Trail parking lot, which is on the right shortly after the road crosses over San Luis Obispo Creek. Parking is free; there are restrooms near the lot entrance.

TRAIL USE
Hike, Run, Bike
LENGTH
4.6 miles, 2.0 hours
VERTICAL FEET
±80
DIFFICULTY
– 1 **2** 3 4 5 +
TRAIL TYPE
Out & Back
SURFACE TYPE
Paved

FEATURES
Handicap Access
Child Friendly
Dogs Allowed
Stream
Beach
Birds
Cool & Shady
Great Views
Photo Opportunity

FACILITIES
Restrooms

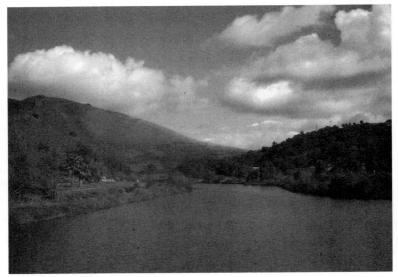

The Bob Jones Trail *runs alongside San Luis Obispo Creek.*

Trail Description

The path begins across the street from the parking lot, otherwise known as the Ontario Road Staging Area. ►1 Look for cross traffic at each of the path's three intersections with neighboring roads, as drivers often speed past on their way to the beach. **Cyclists** should dismount when crossing an intersection. The creek can first be seen at 0.3 mile. At a shady turnout at 0.4 mile, you'll find a couple of benches, which offer nice places to sit and listen to the babbling creek or the resident bird species. At 0.75 mile, the trail runs past a bridge that spans Avila Beach Dr. to the Sycamore Mineral Springs. ►2 At 0.82 mile, a footbridge crosses over a small feeder creek.

The path intersects another busy road, San Luis Bay Dr., at 0.9 mile. ►3 After the first mile, the path passes a private playground and other buildings that make up San Luis Bay Estates. The path runs

 Biking

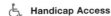 **Handicap Access**

into Blue Heron Dr., ►4 an access road to the gated community at 1.48 mile. Stay to the right, following the road as it follows the creek downstream toward Avila Beach Golf Resort.

Watch for flying golf balls and duck if you hear "fore" while you walk the final leg of the trail. The bike path turns to the left and leaves the access road at 2.16 miles, ►5 passing the 18th tee and crossing a two-lane bridge over the **creek**. Hang a left after the bridge, and reach the trail's official end at 2.3 miles. This is the turnaround. ►6 Return the way you came to reach the parking lot.

◤ Stream

Trail users can continue on the narrow bike path along Avila Beach Dr. to the beach, although it is not considered part of the trail. The beach can be accessed less than 0.25 mile from the trail's official ending.

Notice

City officials were working to extend the path to San Luis Obispo at the time this book was printed. Extending the trail would truly make it run from "city to sea."

The path makes up the final stretch of the popular City to the Sea Half Marathon, which typically runs in October.

🚶	MILESTONES	
►1	0.00	The path begins across the street from the parking lot.
►2	0.75	Trail runs past Sycamore Mineral Springs, located to the left.
►3	0.90	Carefully cross San Luis Bay Dr. and continue down the path.
►4	1.48	The trail merges into Blue Heron Dr.
►5	2.16	The path veers left off the access road by the 18th tee, crossing the two-lane bridge over the creek.
►6	2.30	The turnaround point is where the path ends at Avila Beach Dr.

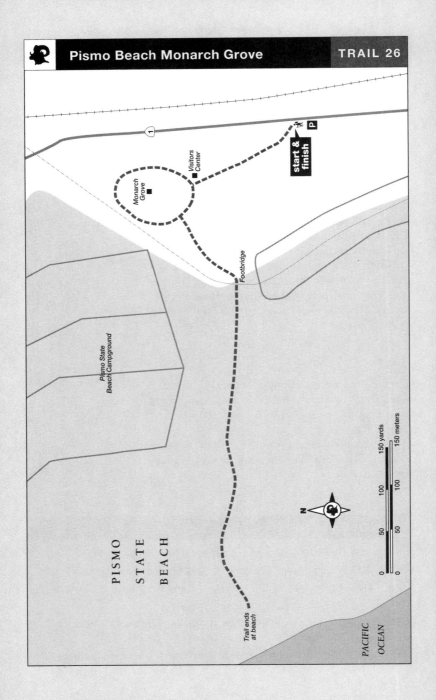

Pismo Beach Monarch Grove — TRAIL 26

Monarch Grove

Visitors Center

start & finish

Footbridge

Pismo State Beach Campground

PISMO STATE BEACH

Trail ends at beach

N

150 yards
150 meters

0   50   100   150

PACIFIC OCEAN

Pismo Beach Monarch Grove

This Pismo Beach trail, which winds through eucalyptus trees that host clusters of butterflies during the wintertime, descends to the stretch of beach south of the pier on a path that parallels a small creek. The monarch colony is one of the largest in the nation, with an average of 100,000 butterflies seeking shelter every year from the winter rains and winds up north.

Best Time

While the trail is a nice, easy stroll all year long, the butterflies don't migrate to the Central Coast until late October and usually remain in the area until February or March. They tend to prefer cool, moist climates, but can't fly when temperatures dip below 55°F. During the season, docents lead daily walks, and a visitors center is usually open from 11 a.m. to 2 p.m. The butterflies are most active during sunny afternoons with little wind.

Finding the Trail

From Hwy. 101 in Pismo Beach, take the Pacific Coast Hwy.–Price exit and travel south for 0.5 mile to Hwy. 1. Hang a right and take the highway south past the pier and look for the grove on the right, after Pismo State Beach Campground and just before the signed city limit to Grover Beach—which is located at 1.5 miles. Park off the side of the road at the dirt turnout and follow the trail to the visitors center. The largest clusters of butterflies can usually be found near the beginning of the trail in the tall eucalyptus trees above.

TRAIL USE
Hike, Run

LENGTH
1.8 miles, 1.0 hour

VERTICAL FEET
±55

DIFFICULTY
− **1** 2 3 4 5 +

TRAIL TYPE
Out & Back

SURFACE TYPE
Dirt, Paved

FEATURES
Child Friendly
Stream
Beach
Fall Color
Wildlife
Birds
Cool & Shady
Great Views
Photo Opportunity
Camping

FACILITIES
Visitors Center
Campground

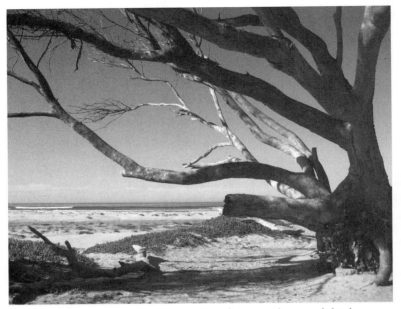

The nature trail *at the Pismo Beach Monarch Butterfly Grove ends at a sandy beach.*

Trail Description

From the parking area, head toward the large eucalyptus trees that line the small creek separating the grove from the nearby campground. The main dirt trail running to the grove meets up with the small visitors center ►1 within 500 feet of the turnout. Follow the trail counterclockwise ►2 under the massive canopy of eucalyptus, watching not squish any resting butterflies on the path.

This is where most of the butterflies hang out, clinging to the leaves and fluttering about the treetops. Bring a set of binoculars to get up-close views of the roosting butterflies, and you'll be surprised at just how many are huddling together for warmth and protection. The trail winds through the heart of the grove and begins to descend to the creek and the beach.

After spending some time watching the butterflies, continue down the main trail to a small
bridge that crosses the creek at 0.25 mile. ▶3 The
creek is a popular hangout for **mallard ducks and**   **Birds**
other coastal waterfowl. Cross the bridge and
make a left on the single track running to the west.
At 0.3 mile, the trail passes another bridge on the
left. Stay straight toward the beach. The trail runs
into the sand at 0.5 mile, ▶4 passing through dunes
anchored by ice plant and various coastal shrubs.

The **beach** offers views of the dunes preserve to   🔄 **Beach**
the south and Pismo Beach Pier, Shell Beach, and

Monarch Facts

The butterflies form dense clusters on the branches of eucalyptus
trees to provide shelter and warmth for the group, protecting the
colony from wind and rain.

The monarchs that visit the Central Coast have a lifespan of
six months, versus six weeks for most common monarchs. This
extended lifespan can be attributed to their unique fat-storing system. The butterflies feed on milkweed, which is poisonous to many
birds. The monarchs that leave in March die off before the colony
returns in the winter.

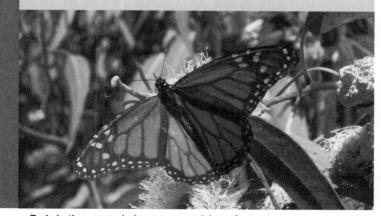

Early in the year *is the best time to watch butterflies.*

Avila Beach to the north. The designated trail disappears beyond the initial set of dunes. Make your own path down to water, ►5 which you'll reach at just under a mile. Return the way you came.

🚶 MILESTONES

►1	0.00	Begin down the main trail to the visitors center.
►2	0.15	Follow the trail counterclockwise through the grove.
►3	0.25	Cross the creek and head left down the dirt single track.
►4	0.50	Stay straight passing a bridge on the left and head down to the water.
►5	0.80	After reaching the water, return the way you came.

Pismo Beach Pier Fishing

It's not as glamorous as fly-fishing for rainbow trout in the Sierra. It doesn't have the same appeal as tackling trophy tuna in the deep sea. But pier fishing at destinations like the Pismo Beach Pier is less expensive, easier to master, and can be equally rewarding—especially when you consider the following:

- Pier anglers regularly catch some of the same sought-after species that charters seek, including halibut, rockfish, and even sharks.

- Pier fishing is free along the Central Coast in most instances.

- No fishing license is required in most cases, because most piers are public property.

- Most Central California piers are open 24 hours a day, which gives anglers a legal means of wetting their lines after work and provides an opportunity to hook up with the large nocturnal feeders that patrol the shallows.

- Plus, it's a lot harder to get seasick on a pier than it is on an afternoon charter boat.

The Pismo Beach Pier is less than 2.0 miles north of the grove off Pomeroy Ave. The top catches at Pismo, along with most San Luis Obispo County piers, are barred surfperch and jacksmelt caught on a Sabiki rig or with shrimp flies.

You can fish the pier supports and breaks for multiple types of surfperch. While trophy catches are rare, the photo wall near the bait shop shows that an occasional bat ray, shovelnose guitarfish, and even a leopard shark aren't out of the question. Pismo Beach is known as the "Clam Capital of the World," but don't use any Pismo clams for bait because it is illegal in most cases to harvest clams at this preserve.

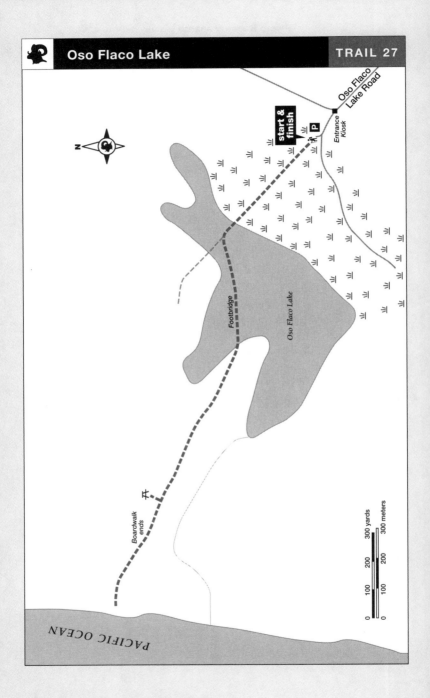

Oso Flaco Lake

TRAIL 27

Oso Flaco Lake Road

start & finish

P

Entrance Kiosk

N

Footbridge

Oso Flaco Lake

Boardwalk ends

300 yards
300 meters

0   100   200   300 yards
0   100   200   300 meters

PACIFIC OCEAN

Oso Flaco Lake

Oso Flaco Lake is the hidden jewel of the South County, tucked away in the Guadalupe–Nipomo Dunes Preserve. A bird-lover's paradise, the lake is just around the corner from a desolate off-road vehicle recreation area and often goes overlooked because of that. Surprisingly enough, this beach lagoon is surrounded by arroyo willows and wax myrtles, making up a riparian corridor that is visited by hundreds of species of birds each year.

Best Time

Oso Flaco Lake is full all year, but the water level is highest—and water clarity is best—in the spring. That is when most of the birds are on hand and the wildflowers along the trail are in full bloom. The trail is open from dawn to dusk.

Finding the Trail

From Hwy. 101 in San Luis Obispo, head south 16 miles to Arroyo Grande and take the Fair Oaks Ave. exit, making a right onto Fair Oaks and following it 0.5 mile to Valley Road. Head left on Valley Road for 1.3 miles and make another left onto Cabrillo Hwy./Hwy. 1, also signed as Cienega St. Follow the highway for 7.8 miles to Oso Flaco Lake Road, turning right and following the road for 3.1 miles to the parking area. There is a $5 parking fee, which can be paid at the kiosk near the park entrance.

TRAIL USE
Hike, Run
LENGTH
2.2 miles, 1.0 hour
VERTICAL FEET
±30
DIFFICULTY
− 1 **2** 3 4 5 +
TRAIL TYPE
Out & Back
SURFACE TYPE
Mixed

FEATURES
Handicap Access
Parking Fee
Child Friendly
Stream
Beach
Lake
Birds
Wildflowers
Wildlife
Great Views

FACILITIES
Restrooms
Picnic Tables

185

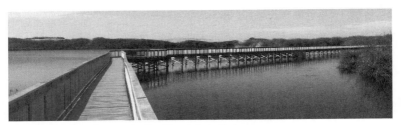

The boardwalk *makes crossing Oso Flaco Lake to the beach a snap.*

Trail Description

From the parking lot, pass the white gate and begin down the access road ►1 beneath the canopy of willows. This thick, shady dune scrub is home to dozens of bird species. The road cuts the lake into two **lagoons**, the largest of which is accessible via a long footbridge located on the left-hand side at 0.3 mile.

 Lake

Make a left and follow the footbridge, ►2 which spans about 0.25 mile, over the larger of the two lagoons. This is where most of the **birds** can be found, floating on the lake's calm surface and ducking in and out of the reeds, searching for food and building their nests. Even to a novice bird-spotter, there are usually dozens of different bird species to see on the lake at any one time.

 Birds

On the tail end of the boardwalk, the park's resident raccoon likes to greet guests in hopes of receiving a little snack. The ranger staff cautions trail users to avoid any contact with the raccoons and in general to avoid feeding the wildlife. You'll find a

NOTES

Thin Bear Lake

In 1979, Don Gaspar de Portola and his group of Spanish explorers were said to have crossed the Santa Maria River and camped here. During their time at the lake, Portola's men killed a thin bear, or "un oso flaco," for which the lake is named.

picnic table is at 0.4 mile, ►3 a nice place for a lunch break if the bugs aren't buzzing about. The walkway reaches the other side of the lake ►4 at 0.5 mile.

A boardwalk, which helps protect the surrounding dune habitat, runs alongside a creek down to the beach. Hikers are encouraged to stay on the trail to prevent damage to the dune vegetation. At 0.88 mile, the trail braches off to another picnic area and restroom facility on the right. Continue down the path toward the sounds of the breaking surf. The boardwalk fades into the sand at 0.7 mile, reappearing and disappearing as the trail shuffles down to the beach.

The trail spits you out at the **beach** at 1.1 miles, ►5 with a view that stretches all the way up to Avila Beach. After soaking up the sun and the sights of this remote beach stretch, return to the parking lot via the boardwalk and access road.

A remote beach is accessible via the trail beyond Oso Flaco Lake, far from the vehicle recreation area to the north.

 Beach

Notice

While the lake is beautiful from above, no swimming is permitted. Also, anglers are warned not to keep fish from the lake as the lake has shown high levels of bacteria and nitrates in years past. Many believe the pollutants stem from runoff from local agricultural fields.

🚶	**MILESTONES**	
►1	0.0	Pass the white gate and follow the access road between the lagoons.
►2	0.3	Make a left onto the footbridge crossing the lake.
►3	0.4	A picnic table and benches offer a spot to sit and watch the birds.
►4	0.5	The footbridge reaches the opposite side of the lake.
►5	1.1	The boardwalk runs into the sand and ends at the beach, which marks the turnaround.

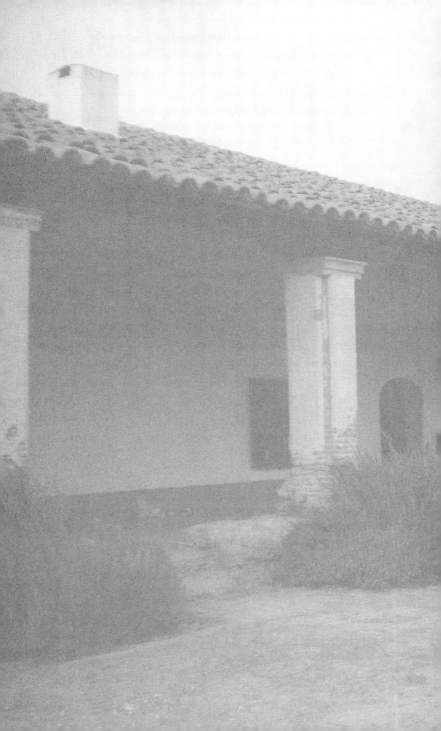

CHAPTER 4

Santa Barbara County

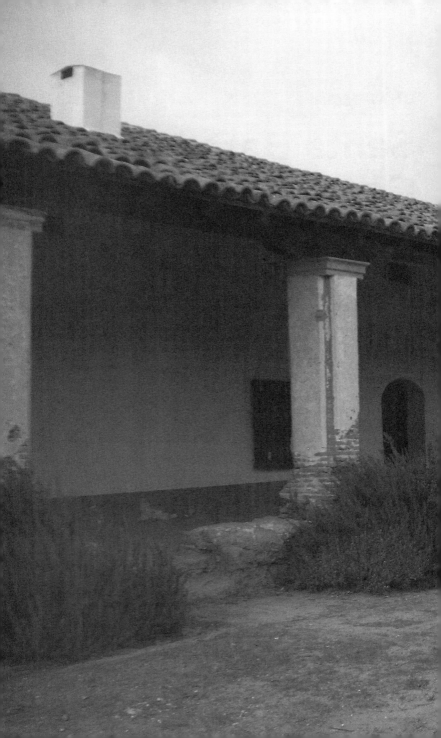

Santa Barbara County

There are so many trails in Santa Barbara County, it's tough to know where to start. If beach trails like the Aniso Trail aren't your thing, there are plenty of other front-country trails that can get your heart racing. La Purisima Mission offers a historic network of trails that explorers and missionaries followed hundreds of years ago. But if history isn't your favorite subject, try biology: Study the plant and animal life at the base of Nojoqui Falls and atop Gaviota Peak.

Once you've tested the front-country trails, head for the Santa Barbara foothills where Inspiration Point, Seven Falls, Montecito Overlook, and San Ysidro Trail will help you get away from it all. Continue inland along East Camino Cielo, and you'll run into Blue Canyon and the Santa Ynez River Valley.

Tremendous views of the valley can be had along the remaining trails, whether you're perched high above the valley at Knapp's Castle or Figueroa Lookout, or smack-dab in the middle of it at the Gibraltar Reservoir.

Permits and Maps

Most of the backcountry trails in Santa Barbara County are located within the Los Padres National Forest. A National Forest Adventure Pass is required for many Los Padres hikes, including those in the Santa Ynez River Recreation Area. A pass can be purchased at ranger stations and area sporting goods retailers, including Big 5 in Santa Barbara. The $30 passes can also be ordered by calling (909) 382-2622.

View Los Padres National Forest maps at www.fs.fed.us/r5/forestvisitormaps/lospadres or purchase them at www.nationalforeststore.com. For more information, contact the Los Padres ranger station in Goleta at (805) 968-6640.

There is a parking fee at La Purisima Mission. A map of the many trails on the mission grounds can be purchased at the entrance gate. The Aniso Trailhead is at Refugio State Beach, where there is a day-use fee. A park map is available at the entrance kiosk.

Overleaf and opposite: *La Purisima Mission was the 11th of California's 21 Spanish missions.*

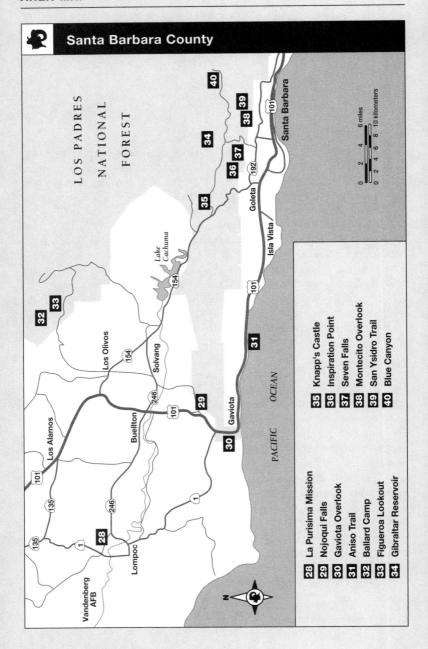

Santa Barbara County

LOS PADRES
NATIONAL
FOREST

Lake
Cachuma

Los Olivos
Solvang
Buellton
Los Alamos
Lompoc
Vandenberg AFB

Goleta
Isla Vista
Santa Barbara

PACIFIC OCEAN

Gaviota

28 La Purisima Mission
29 Nojoqui Falls
30 Gaviota Overlook
31 Aniso Trail
32 Ballard Camp
33 Figueroa Lookout
34 Gibraltar Reservoir

35 Knapp's Castle
36 Inspiration Point
37 Seven Falls
38 Montecito Overlook
39 San Ysidro Trail
40 Blue Canyon

0 2 4 6 miles
0 2 4 6 8 10 kilometers

N

TRAIL FEATURE TABLE

Santa Barbara County

TRAIL	Difficulty	Length	Type	USES & ACCESS	TERRAIN	FLORA & FAUNA	OTHER
28	2	3.8	Out & Back	Hiking, Horses, Running, Biking, Child Friendly, Fee, Dogs Allowed	Meadow	Fall Color, Birds, Wildlife	Historic Interest
29	1	1.0	Out & Back	Hiking, Running, Child Friendly, Dogs Allowed	River or Stream, Waterfall	Fall Color, Birds	Secluded, Cool and Shady
30	4	3.25	Out & Back	Hiking, Horses, Running, Biking	River or Stream, Mountain	Wildflowers, Birds, Wildlife	Great Views, Steep, Secluded, Photo Opportunity
31	3	5.0	Out & Back	Hiking, Running, Biking, Child Friendly, Handicap Access, Fee, Dogs Allowed	River or Stream, Beach, Canyon		
32	5	4.6	Out & Back	Hiking, Horses, Running, Biking, Permit Required	River or Stream, Canyon	Wildflowers, Fall Color, Birds, Wildlife	Great Views, Steep, Secluded, Camping, Cool and Shady
33	5	4.45	Out & Back	Hiking, Horses, Running, Biking, Permit Required	River or Stream, Mountain	Wildflowers, Fall Color, Birds, Wildlife	Great Views, Steep, Camping
34	5	6.0	Out & Back	Hiking, Horses, Running, Biking, Permit Required, Dogs Allowed	River or Stream, Lake, Canyon, Mountain	Wildflowers, Birds	
35	1	1.0	Out & Back	Hiking, Running, Biking, Child Friendly, Permit Required	Lake, Canyon	Wildflowers, Fall Color, Birds, Wildlife	Historic Interest, Great Views, Photo Opportunity
36	3	3.6	Out & Back	Hiking, Running, Biking, Dogs Allowed	River or Stream, Waterfall, Canyon	Fall Color, Birds	Great Views, Photo Opportunity
37	4	2.6	Out & Back	Hiking, Running, Dogs Allowed	River or Stream, Waterfall, Canyon	Fall Color, Birds	Great Views, Photo Opportunity
38	4	3.0	Out & Back	Hiking, Horses, Running, Biking, Permit Required, Dogs Allowed	River or Stream, Mountain	Wildflowers, Birds, Wildlife	Great Views, Steep, Secluded, Photo Opportunity
39	5	4.0	Point-to-Point	Hiking, Horses, Running, Biking, Permit Required, Dogs Allowed	River or Stream, Waterfall, Canyon, Mountain	Wildflowers, Birds, Wildlife	Great Views, Steep, Photo Opportunity
40	3	3.2	Out & Back	Hiking, Running, Biking, Child Friendly, Permit Required, Dogs Allowed	River or Stream, Canyon	Wildflowers, Birds	Geologic Interest, Secluded, Camping

Legend

USES & ACCESS
- Hiking
- Horses
- Running
- Biking
- Child Friendly
- Handicap Access
- $ Fee
- Permit Required
- Dogs Allowed

TYPE
- Loop
- Out & Back
- Point-to-Point

DIFFICULTY
- 1 2 3 4 5 +
- less   more

TERRAIN
- River or Stream
- Waterfall
- Lake
- Beach
- Tide Pools
- Canyon
- Mountain
- Meadow

FLORA & FAUNA
- Wildflowers
- Fall Color
- Birds
- Wildlife

FEATURES
- Historic Interest
- Geologic Interest
- Great Views
- Steep
- Secluded
- Cool and Shady
- Camping
- Photo Opportunity

Santa Barbara County

Ballard Camp 217

The trail to Ballard Camp is often overlooked because it does not have a clear-cut parking area or designated trailhead sign. These things make it that much more peaceful. This remote backcountry hike passes some of the most spectacular wildflower displays the Central Coast has to offer before descending to the canyon floor, where a spring-fed stream runs past an old cabin site.

TRAIL 32

Hike, Run, Bike, Horse
4.6 miles, 3.0 hours
Out & Back
Difficulty: 1 2 3 4 **5**

Figueroa Lookout 221

The best lookout point in the Figueroa Mountain Recreation Area, Figueroa Lookout can be reached via a fire-road trail that presents a challenging ride for mountain bikers. Be sure to make a brief stop at Pino Alto Nature Trail along the way.

TRAIL 33

Hike, Run, Bike, Horse
4.45 miles, 3.0 hours
Out & Back
Difficulty: 1 2 3 4 **5**

Gibraltar Reservoir 227

While the Red Rock Trail often gets bombarded by hikers during the spring and summer months, this fire road trail leading to the crystal-clear Gibraltar Reservoir sees little action. It can be a demanding climb for mountain bikers and hikers alike.

TRAIL 34

Hike, Run, Bike, Horse
6.0 miles, 3.0 hours
Out & Back
Difficulty: 1 2 3 4 **5**

Knapp's Castle 233

Set high above the Santa Ynez River Valley, the old site of Knapp's Castle offers outstanding views of the Santa Ynez River and the neighboring reservoir. Brick arches, entryways, and chimneys are all that remain of George Knapp's mountain lodge.

TRAIL 35

Hike, Run, Bike
1.0 mile, 0.5 hour
Out & Back
Difficulty: **1** 2 3 4 5

TRAIL 36

Hike, Run, Bike
3.6 miles, 1.5 hours
Out & Back
Difficulty: 1 2 **3** 4 5

Inspiration Point. 239

An exhilarating climb up to one of Santa Barbara's best vantage points, Inspiration Point offers unfathomable views of the city, ocean, and the islands across the channel. Along the way, the trail follows Mission Creek, skirting its many pools, which are popular with swimmers in the summer.

TRAIL 37

Hike, Run
2.6 miles, 1.5 hours
Out & Back
Difficulty: 1 2 3 **4** 5

Seven Falls. 243

Starting out along the same route as the Inspiration Point Trail, the single track to Seven Falls veers off the beaten path at Mission Creek and follows it upstream to a series of falls that spill from one pool to another. The lower pools are popular with swimmers in the early summer, but get away from the lower stretches of Mission Creek and the trail is as technical as it is challenging.

TRAIL 38

Hike, Run, Bike, Horse
3.0 miles, 2.0 hours
Out & Back
Difficulty: 1 2 3 **4** 5

Montecito Overlook 247

This trail is the quickest way to the Montecito Overlook area, which is perched 2,500 feet above Santa Barbara County coast. The hike back up the Cold Spring Trail, however, is anything but a piece of cake and presents a taxing climb back to the parking area. There's also a side trip to Montecito Peak for those who are looking for a real climb.

San Ysidro Trail

TRAIL 39

Hike, Run, Bike, Horse
4.0 miles, 2.0 hours
Point-to-Point
Difficulty: 1 2 3 4 **5**

The San Ysidro Trail is listed as a point-to-point hike because its 3,000-foot elevation change makes it too grueling to treat as an out-and-back hike. It's used primarily by mountain bikers as a fun, technical downhill. Along the way, the trail passes numerous feeder creeks and offers great vantage points for viewing the coast.

Blue Canyon

TRAIL 40

Hike, Run, Bike
3.2 miles, 1.5 hours
Out & Back
Difficulty: 1 2 **3** 4 5

This Santa Ynez River Valley hike runs along Forbush Creek and passes grove after grove on the way to the Upper Blue Canyon Camp. The trail is named for the bluish-colored serpentine that lines the canyon.

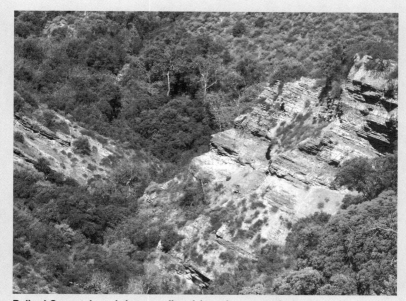

Ballard Camp *is located along a small creek beneath a canopy of oaks.*

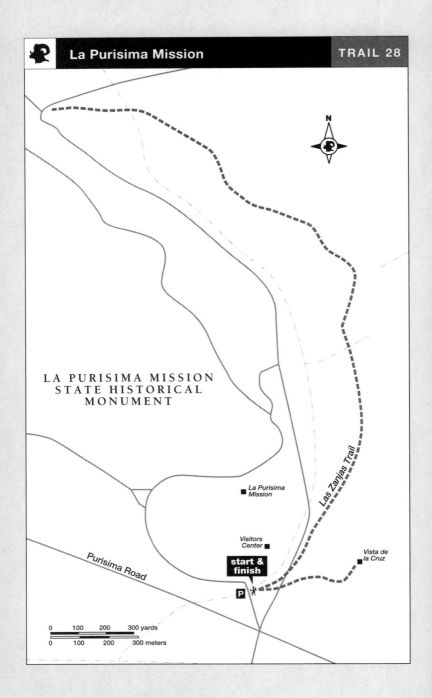

La Purisima Mission — TRAIL 28

N

LA PURISIMA MISSION
STATE HISTORICAL
MONUMENT

Las Zanjas Trail

La Purisima
Mission

Visitors
Center

Vista de
la Cruz

start &
finish

Purisima Road

P

0   100   200   300 yards
0   100   200   300 meters

La Purisima Mission

The 11th of California's 21 Spanish missions, La Purisima in Lompoc offers many of the same trails explorers and mission residents followed in the 1700s and 1800s. La Purisima is home to some of the best horseback riding trails on the Central Coast, although many of the routes go overlooked because they make up the backdrop to this historic landmark.

Best Time

La Purisima's trails are open daily from 9 a.m. to 5 p.m., except for Thanksgiving, Christmas, and New Year's Day. Also, the trails may be closed to the public during the rainy season to help protect them from damage and erosion.

Finding the Trail

From Hwy. 101 in Buellton, take Hwy. 246 west for 14 miles. Take a right on Purisima Road for less than 1.0 mile, and the La Purisima State Historic Park entrance is on the right. There is an entrance fee of $4. A map of the mission grounds and its trails costs $1 and is recommended for trail users because many of the single tracks are unmarked. There are more than 1,800 acres and 25 miles of trails within the park. This particular hike follows the main Las Zanjas Trail through the heart of the mission's interior and finishes with a short climb up the Vista de La Cruz, thus following two of the most popular trails for hikers, mountain bikers, and equestrians.

TRAIL USE
Hike, Run, Bike, Horse
LENGTH
3.8 miles, 2.0 hours
VERTICAL FEET
±100
DIFFICULTY
− 1 **2** 3 4 5 +
TRAIL TYPE
Out & Back
SURFACE TYPE
Dirt

FEATURES
Entrance Fee
Child Friendly
Dogs Allowed
Meadow
Fall Color
Birds
Wildlife
Historic

FACILITIES
Restrooms
Picnic Tables
Water
Phone
Visitors Center

Trail Description

The mission was founded on December 8, 1787, by Father Fermin Lasuen. Portions of the mission grounds, including the livestock pens and pastures, are still in use today.

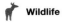 **Wildlife**

 Great Views

The Las Zanjas Trailhead is near the main parking lot; follow the main fire road behind the visitors center and continue north toward the Spring House. ►1 Early in the hike, you'll pass the start of the La Artemisila Trail. Stay straight until you reach the Spring House at 0.5 mile. ►2 Water from springs and a reservoir that were nearby was once channeled to the Spring House, where it was then filtered through sand. Today, the water is shipped through clay pipes to the fountain in the Mission Garden.

You'll get a better look at the mission's aqueduct system as you continue north along the fire road. To the west of the trail sits a field that was once the main beneficiary of the mission's elaborate irrigation system. Today, the field is a popular spot for **deer**, **quail**, and even the occasional **kangaroo rat**. ►3 Continue down the fire road and stay left where the trail splits at 1.4 miles. The turnaround is just ahead, at 1.6 miles. Return to the parking lot the way you came.

At the parking lot, you'll see the Vista de La Cruz (Landmark Cross) Trailhead, ►4 not far from the Las Zanjas Trailhead. This path is a moderate climb that starts behind the visitors center and rises 0.3 mile to the cross above. ►5 From the cross, you can **look down upon the bell tower, main church, residence buildings, and garden**. Walk back down the Vista de La Cruz Trail to the parking lot, rounding out your 3.8-mile hike.

Notice

La Purisima is one of the few state parks that allow dogs on its trails. Dogs are permitted on the trails if they are kept on a leash.

MILESTONES

▶1　0.0　Follow the fire road that runs behind the visitors center to the north.

▶2　0.5　The trail runs past the Spring House where water was collected for irrigation.

▶3　0.8　Continue down the fire road, which runs parallel to the aqueduct running to the Spring House.

▶4　1.4　Stay left at the fork in the trail and reach the turnaround spot shortly thereafter.

▶5　3.2　Return the way you came and find the Vista de La Cruz hike, a self-explanatory, half-mile hike to the cross above.

OPTIONS

Other Purisima Mission Trails

Because La Purisima Mission State Park covers 1,800 acres and has 25 miles of trails, there are far too many trail options to list. Many of the trails are unmarked, which make purchasing a map for $1 and bringing along a portable GPS unit both good ideas.

Some notable trails for optional hikes are El Noque, Arca de Agua, El Camino Real, and Cuclillo de Tierra.

- The trail to El Noque is a 0.24-mile hike that runs to the mission's hide-tanning vats and is popular with trail runners, who combine El Noque with other trails.

- Arca de Agua, or the reservoir, is a 0.64-mile path that is popular with equestrians and passes through a wide range of plant communities ranging from wetland to chaparral.

- El Camino Real, or the royal highway, is a 1.0-mile hike believed to be a portion of the original trail between the missions and presidios of early California.

- Cuclillo de Tierra, or the roadrunner, is another popular trail run or ride that follows the service road on the upper loop.

Additional paths and trails weave in and out of the interior of the mission and its historic buildings and gardens.

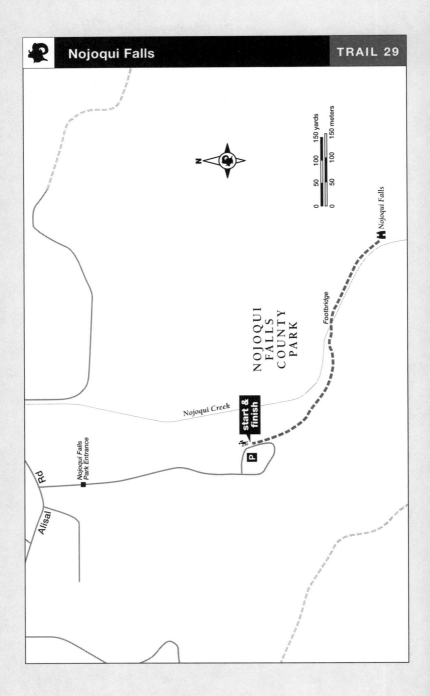

NOJOQUI
FALLS
COUNTY
PARK

Nojoqui Falls

Footbridge

Nojoqui Creek

start & finish

P

Nojoqui Falls
Park Entrance

Rd

Alisal

0   50   100   150 yards
0   50   100   150 meters

N

Nojoqui Falls

At first glance, Nojoqui Falls County Park looks like your average city park with sports fields, barbecue grills, and group picnic areas. But tucked away toward the back of this Gaviota Pass-area park is a local secret—an 80-foot-high waterfall tumbling down a sandstone cliff that's painted green with Venus maidenhair ferns. This short but sweet hike offers a quick glance at one of Santa Barbara County's few year-round waterfalls and is a nice, easy stroll for all ages.

Best Time

The waterfall is most impressive after the rainy season, although the trail is a relatively flat, comfortable hike all year because it passes almost entirely through the shade. Nojoqui Creek usually runs throughout the year, although the waterfall can lose some of its luster by fall.

Finding the Trail

The turnoff for Nojoqui Falls is located about 2.0 miles north of the Gaviota Pass tunnel on the east side of Hwy. 101 (about 40 miles north of Santa Barbara). Make a right on Old Coast Hwy. and follow the stretch of old highway for just under a mile before making a left on Alisal Road. The park is on the right in another mile. Drive through the park, following the signs to the clearly marked trailhead at the end of the loop.

TRAIL USE
Hike, Run
LENGTH
1.0 mile, 0.5 hour
VERTICAL FEET
±98
DIFFICULTY
− **1** 2 3 4 5 +
TRAIL TYPE
Out & Back
SURFACE TYPE
Mixed

FEATURES
Child Friendly
Dogs Allowed
Stream
Waterfall
Fall Color
Birds
Cool & Shady
Secluded

FACILITIES
Restrooms
Picnic Tables
Water

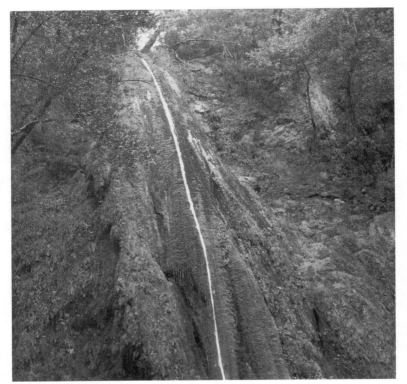

Nojoqui Falls *slows to a trickle during the summer months.*

Trail Description

The trailhead is past the parking loop, from where the trail follows Nojoqui Creek upstream to the base of the falls. Nearly the entire trail is in the shade, which makes this a breeze of a hike that's **appealing for both children and their grandparents**. It also is a popular destination for trail runners looking for a quick 1.0-mile jog. You'll come to benches within the first 400 feet of the hike, which make a nice picnic spot. ▶1

At 0.15 mile, ▶2 you can hear the gargle of the **creek**. (After a good rain, it can actually be heard

 Child Friendly

 Stream

from the parking lot as it tumbles on down through historic Nojoqui Falls Ranch.)

The trail crosses a first bridge at 0.25 mile. After the small footbridge, 20 steps lead up to another small bridge. ▶3 This is the portion of the trail that is not handicapped accessible, although its lower portions are paved, and suited for wheelchairs. At this point, you can hear the falls, which are just around the bend, at an elevation of just 960 feet.

While there is little wildlife along the trail's lower reaches, aside from the occasional gray squirrel, there are many species of **birds** that call the sycamores above home, including noisy acorn woodpeckers and some migratory species.

🐦 **Birds**

The **waterfall** is located at 0.5 mile, ▶4 beyond a pair of signs that explain how Nojoqui Creek was able to cut a steep-walled gorge into the fractured shale of the Jalama Formation, which can't be accessed publicly but is located on the upper reaches of the creek. The cascade runs over where shale and sandstone converge and, as the sign notes, "where rock grows over time." Because the waterfall creates calcium and magnesium deposits on the cliff, the rock is actually growing outward instead of eroding. Venus maidenhair ferns grow alongside the falls, thriving on the calcium-rich cliff.

🔲 **Waterfall**

After feeling the mist of the waterfall, retrace your steps to the parking lot.

🚶 **MILESTONES**

▶1	0.00	From the parking lot, follow the trailhead signs past a picnic area.
▶2	0.15	The trail follows Nojoqui Creek upstream all the way to the falls.
▶3	0.25	After a small footbridge, hikers will encounter 20 short steps leading to another bridge.
▶4	0.50	The falls is at 0.5 mile, which makes it an even 1.0-mile trip when you return the way you came.

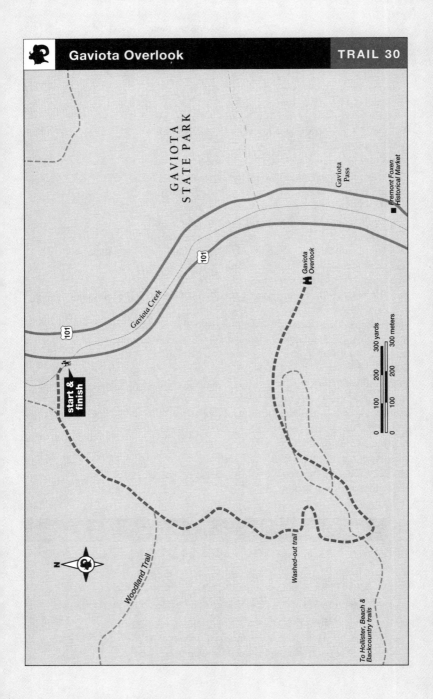

Gaviota Overlook

TRAIL 30

GAVIOTA STATE PARK

Gaviota Pass

■ Fremont Foxen
Historical Market

101

Gaviota Creek

101

Gaviota Overlook

start & finish

300 yards

300 meters

200

200

100

100

0

0

N

Woodland Trail

Washed-out trail

To Hollister, Beach &
Backcountry trails

Gaviota Overlook

The best part about this secluded, somewhat steep hike to the ridgeline—next to the amazing views from the ridgeline—is the fact that it's a freebie. While many of the hikes through the rolling backcountry of 2,700-acre Gaviota State Park will require a day-use fee, this particular trailhead offers free access and the same great views of the park.

Best Time

Because the trail follows an old fire road, the path remains relatively clear throughout the year, despite seeing little use during the winter and spring months. Portions of the trail have washed out, so use caution when hiking during the rainy season, when strong winds can make the ridgeline portion of the trail miserable. The trail can get hot along the grasslands and ridgeline in the summer months.

Finding the Trail

Despite being within a few feet of the southbound lane of Hwy. 101, this trail is tricky to find. The trailhead is north of Gaviota Pass, about 10 miles south of Buellton. Take Hwy. 101 south past the Hwy. 1/Lompoc exit and look for the blue sign that notes REST AREA, 1.0 MILE. It is important to remain in the slow lane at this point, slowing down and signaling for the turnout to fend off tailgaters. The turnout by the trail's entrance is just past the blue sign, on the opposite side of the concrete bridge that follows. If you miss the turnoff, you'll have to drive down to the Gaviota State Park exit and turn around. When

TRAIL USE
Hike, Run, Bike, Horse
LENGTH
3.25 miles, 2.0 hours
VERTICAL FEET
±600
DIFFICULTY
− 1 2 3 **4** 5 +
TRAIL TYPE
Out & Back
SURFACE TYPE
Dirt

FEATURES
Mountain
Steep
Stream
Birds
Wildflowers
Wildlife
Great Views
Photo Opportunity
Secluded

you reach the turnoff, park off to the side, without blocking the gate.

Trail Description

 Stream

Look for trail notices at the gate before you start the climbing on this forgotten-about ranch road. The trail passes year-round **Gaviota Creek** along with a handful of seasonal creeks along the lower portions of the trail. ▶1 By 0.5 mile, the sights and sounds of a hectic Hwy. 101 take a back seat to the upland oak woodlands, grasslands, and chaparral of the park. This trail, popular with bird-watchers, winds through many different habitats for the region's diverse bird species. The Woodland Trailhead can be found at 0.55 mile; stay straight. ▶2 A portion of the trail is washed out at 0.85 mile—use the single track to the right to avoid the washout. ▶3 Immediately after completing the first mile, you'll pass the start of the Hollister Trail, and the end of the Beach to Backcountry Trail, which heads uphill from the main park near the beach. Stay left ▶4 and continue on the main Outlook Trail up to the ridge. At 1.75 miles, marked by a set of radio towers, the trail ends. ▶5 At the top, some 827 feet above sea level, trail users are greeted with **sweeping views** of the Gaviota coast, including the beach-access park below, Gaviota Pass, and, on clear days, panoramic shots of the islands across the channel. To the east lies 2,458-foot Gaviota Peak. Return the way you came.

Great Views

Beach Access

NOTES

Gaviota State Park offers beach access to the cove and pier, popular spots for anglers, divers, and surfers. There is a day-use fee for beach users. Camping, consisting of 41 first-come, first-served campsites, is available at the main park. Call Gaviota State Park (805) 968-1033 directly for more information.

MILESTONES

▶1   0.00   Trail follows a ranch road and passes Gaviota Creek and other streams.

▶2   0.50   Continue straight and pass Woodland Trailhead.

▶3   0.60   Take the single track to avoid the washed-out portion of the main fire road.

▶4   1.10   Continue left, past turnoffs to the Hollister and Beach to Backcountry trails.

▶5   1.75   Trail ends at the towers, which mark the turnaround.

Other Trails

OPTIONS

Gaviota State Park has countless dirt fire roads and trails that weave in and out of its oak woodland and chaparral backcountry. Pick up a map at the park entrance, which is about 2.0 miles south of the Gaviota Overlook Trailhead off Hwy. 101.

• The Woodland Trail, which starts 0.55 mile into the Gaviota Overlook Trail, climbs a dirt single track for another 0.6 mile up to 1.5-mile Hollister Trail and its peak at 968 feet.

• The Hollister Trail turns to the north and meets up with the Yucca Trail (1.0 mile) and the Las Cruces Trail (1.1 miles).

• The Las Cruces Trail tracks back to the Ortega Trail (0.7 mile), which completes the loop back to the beginning of the Gaviota Overlook Trail.

• Another popular hike on this northern side of the 101 is the Beach to Backcountry Trail, a 1.75-mile path from the beach at the state park up to the Overlook Trail.

Across Hwy. 101, trailheads to Gaviota Hot Springs and Gaviota Peak in the Los Padres National Forest can be accessed via a park entrance about 2.5 miles north of the main park. Take Hwy. 101 north to the Lompoc exit and turn right at the stop sign. Follow the frontage road back south to the trailhead parking area. From this trailhead, hikers have access to the Tunnel View (1.1 miles), the Gaviota Hot Springs (0.7 mile), the Gaviota Peak (3.2 miles), and the Trespass (0.8 mile) trails.

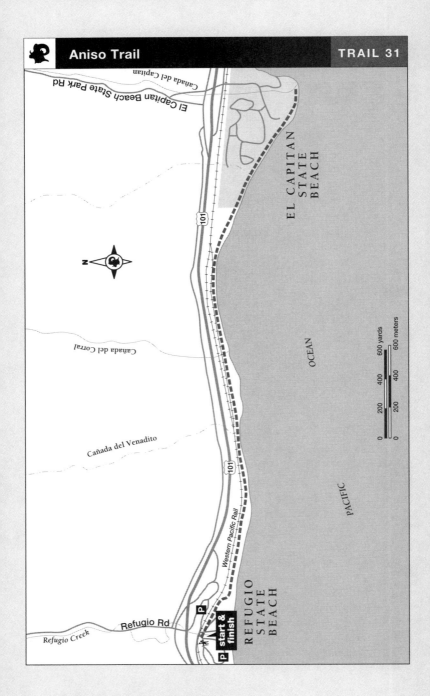

Aniso Trail

TRAIL 31

El Capitan Beach State Park Rd

Cañada del Capitan

EL CAPITAN STATE BEACH

101

N

Cañada del Corral

Cañada del Venadito

OCEAN

0   200   400   600 yards

0   200   400   600 meters

101

PACIFIC

Western Pacific Rail

REFUGIO STATE BEACH

Refugio Rd

Refugio Creek

P

P

start & finish

Aniso Trail

Better known as the Refugio to El Capitán bike path in Goleta, the Aniso Trail is said to be an old route the Chumash used to reach what is now the Santa Barbara coast. *Aniso* is a Chumash word for "gull." The California gull, which is gray, white, and black and easily identified by its yellow, red-tipped bill, is the resident bird of the Goleta coast.

The Aniso Trail is a paved, two-lane path that borders the seaside cliffs between one state beach and another. It is an easy-to-maneuver path that has little elevation gain, so it is popular with cyclists and families who stay at the bookend campgrounds. It is a nice change for runners who are wary about uneven backcountry trails but get tired of running through street traffic. The Aniso Trail is an ideal getaway, offering a 5.0-mile run without the traffic and with coastal views that make the Pacific Coast Hwy. famous.

Best Time

A hike for all seasons, this bluff-top path offers the best coastal views on clear, sunny days. Many beachgoers like to hike back along the beach during a negative tide, so check the tide tables before the return hike.

Finding the Trail

Refugio State Beach is about 25 miles west of Santa Barbara, on the west side of Hwy. 101. Although the beach is west of Santa Barbara, you take Hwy. 101 north to get there. Refugio State Beach is 50 miles

TRAIL USE
Hike, Run, Bike

LENGTH
5.0 miles, 3.0 hours

VERTICAL FEET
±50

DIFFICULTY
– 1 2 **3** 4 5 +

TRAIL TYPE
Out & Back

SURFACE TYPE
Paved

FEATURES
Handicap Access
Parking Fee
Child Friendly
Dogs Allowed
Canyon
Stream
Beach

FACILITIES
Restrooms
Picnic Tables
Water
Phone
Campground

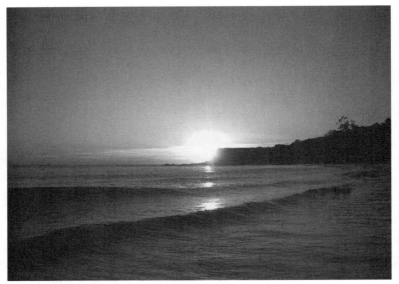

Refugio Beach *is home to some spectacular sunsets.*

south of Santa Maria, accessible via Hwy. 101 south. Free parking is available under the highway overpass; there is a day-use fee for parking in the park. The trailhead is located where the road into the park forks to the separate camping areas.

Trail Description

The trail starts near Refugio Creek ▶1 and heads east to El Capitán, passing the Bouchard camping area and leaving Refugio State Beach within the first 0.25 mile.

At 0.23 mile ▶2 is a kiosk explaining the origin of the trail's name. From here, the trail levels out, running between the railroad tracks and beach for nearly the entire stretch. There is a fence between much of the trail and the tracks, but trail users are still encouraged to pay close attention to children and to avoid the railroad area and cliff edges.

Fishing along the Beaches

While many anglers in Santa Barbara County stick to deep-sea fishing off the Channel Islands or freshwater bass fishing at Lake Cachuma, surf fishing is becoming quite popular along the remote beaches between Refugio and El Capitán. The most common catch for wader-clad anglers along this stretch is surfperch, which often bunch up in schools along the breaks. Silver, calico, redtail, and walleye surfperch can all be found on the Central Coast, although barred surfperch make up most of the bites.

Surfperch can be caught on everything from mud shrimp to sand crabs and plastic grubs that resemble the saltwater species these schools feed on. The most popular plastic bait seems to be motor oil grubs with gold flakes. Fly-anglers catch fish on streamers, various shrimp flies, and always have a chance to hook up with halibut, stripers, and even steelhead.

Most anglers stick to spinning reels and 8-foot-plus surf rods. Common setups are 10- to 20-pound test line; leaders with size 2–6 hooks and pyramid weights are also common. But the size and weight of tackle should correlate with conditions such as the drift, tide, and wave height and frequency. Although surfperch can be caught all day long, it's best to work breaks in the early morning when the conditions are calm.

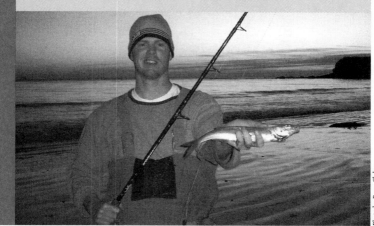

Photo by Beau Clyburn

Jacksmelt and surfperch *are the most common catches by surf anglers.*

At 0.6 mile, the trail passes a tall palm, one of many planted at Refugio. At the 1.0-mile mark, the trail strays away from the railroad tracks and runs right along the cliff edge. Also known as Cañada Del Venadito, ►3 this part might be the **best lookout** between the beaches—you can gaze out across the channel to Santa Rosa and Santa Cruz islands. At 1.5 miles, you'll come to a water tunnel ►4 through which runoff from the Santa Ynez Mountains reaches the beach.

The path reaches El Capitán in just over 2.0 miles. ►5 It continues for another 0.5 mile to Cañada del Capitán, ►6 where a stairway provides access from the bluffs to the sandy beach below. The sycamore and oak trees that line El Capitán Creek provide a **shady resting spot** before the return trip back to Refugio. Some trail users return to Refugio via the beach if tides allow, although the best bet is to return via the same paved path, as creek crossings and **tide pools** can make for a challenging route back.

Notice

There are several spurs off the paved path that cross the railroad tracks and lead down to the beach and tide pool area. Hike with caution if you must leave the path. Remember, there is a stairway at El Capitán State Beach.

There are campgrounds at both beaches, along with public restrooms and snack bars that are usually open during the summer months.

Great Views

Cool & Shady

Tide Pools

⚐ MILESTONES

▶1   0.00   Start near the trailhead at Refugio Creek.

▶2   0.23   Reach kiosk explaining the trail's name.

▶3   1.00   Pass Cañada Del Venadito.

▶4   1.50   Continue past the water tunnel.

▶5   2.10   Enter El Capitán State Park.

▶6   2.50   Turn around at Cañada del Capitán.

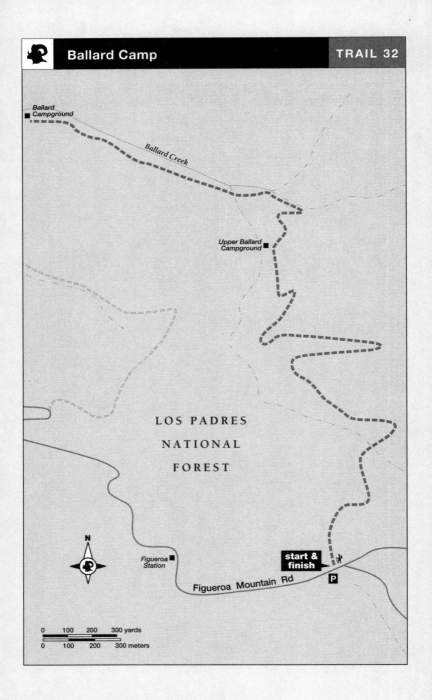

Ballard Camp

TRAIL 32

Ballard Campground

Ballard Creek

Upper Ballard Campground

LOS PADRES

NATIONAL

FOREST

N

Figueroa Station

start & finish

P

Figueroa Mountain Rd

0   100   200   300 yards

0   100   200   300 meters

Ballard Camp

Ballard Camp Trail, part of the La Jolla Trail, is a steep single track that descends quickly to the canyon floor, where a spring-fed stream runs past an old California Conservation Corps cabin and a pair of campsites. It's an easy hike down but is one heck of a hike back up. This easy-to-miss trail is in the Figueroa Mountain Recreation Area about 30 minutes north of Los Olivos and is open to hiking, horseback riding, and mountain biking.

Best Time

The spring is the best season to tackle this trail because of the warming weather and blooming wildflowers. You may see snow in the winter and 100°F temperatures in the summer, although at this elevation, the canyon floor is shaded well by the tall pines and forest.

Finding the Trail

From Santa Barbara, take Hwy. 101 to the Hwy. 154/ Cachuma Lake exit. Head northwest on Hwy. 154/ San Marcos Pass past the Cachuma Recreation Area. When you reach the small town of Los Olivos, make a right on Figueroa Mountain Road and follow the winding road for 12 miles to the Figueroa ranger station. The trailhead, easy to miss because it is marked only by a brown trail marker, is 0.5 mile past the ranger station, across from the turnoff to Tunnel Road. Park in the dirt turnout opposite Tunnel Road and avoid blocking the driveway. An Adventure Pass is required. The trailhead is indicated by the plastic Los Padres National Forest marker.

TRAIL USE
Hike, Run, Bike, Horse
LENGTH
4.6 miles, 3.0 hours
VERTICAL FEET
±835
DIFFICULTY
– 1 2 3 4 **5** +
TRAIL TYPE
Out & Back
SURFACE TYPE
Dirt

FEATURES
Permit Required
Canyon
Steep
Stream
Fall Color
Birds
Wildflowers
Wildlife
Cool & Shady
Great Views
Camping
Secluded

Trail Description

 Steep

The first 1.5 mile of the trail is the fun part—**it descends more than 800 feet**. The single track starts off at 3,328 feet ►1 and races through wonderful wildflower displays, with blue lupines, chocolate lilies, and golden poppies dotting the upper meadow areas in the spring.

The trail crosses an intermittent stream at 0.2 mile ►2 and continues carving through blooming hillsides to a gorgeous lookout over the Santa Ynez Valley at 0.8 mile. ►3 This is where the trail really starts to descend. From just before the 1.0-mile mark to the **canyon floor**, the trail endures five sharp switchbacks to Upper Ballard Camp over a half-mile stretch.

Canyon

The canyon floor is at 1.5 miles. ►4 The upper camp is just around the bend, near the babbling seasonal creek. Follow the creek downstream for

Other Area Trails

OPTIONS

There are dozens of hikes in the Figueroa Mountain region. The Ballard Camp Trail is one of the least-traveled routes, although it is a rewarding trip for backpackers. The Davy Brown Trail is probably the most popular path in the region, running 3.0 miles and following the creek to an old mine shaft and miner's cabin.

There are two widely popular trails along Manzana Creek, which is closed to mountain bikes. The Upper Manzana Creek Trail is a 14-mile stretch that heads east up the creek from Nira Campground. The Lower Manzana Creek Trail is an 8.0-mile jaunt northwest to the Sisquoc River.

Some other Figueroa trails to consider include Zaca Peak (2.5 miles), Sulphur Springs (4.0 miles), Catway (2.5 miles), Willow Springs (2.0 miles), Willow Spur (1.0 mile), Munch Canyon Trail (3.5 miles), White Rock Trail (2.0 miles), McKinley Trail (10.0 miles), and Sunset Valley Trail (2.0 miles). Another popular hike, this one to the Pino Alto Nature Trail and Figueroa Lookout, is covered next, in Trail 33.

0.2 mile to the **camping site**, ►5 which is marked by the remains of an old cabin and some usable fire pits. Check current fire restrictions within the Los Padres National Forest, as this area was hit hard by the Zaca Fire in the summer of 2007.

⚠ Camping

Watch for poison oak, as the trail continues alongside the creek for another 0.6 mile to lower Ballard Camp and Ballard Creek, ►6 a popular Boy Scout camp that marks the end of the journey at 2.3 miles and an elevation of 2,493 feet. Return the way you came, taking your time, as the second half of the trail is a grueling climb that ascends 800 feet over the final 1.5 miles.

Notice

Note that some maps refer to Ballard Camp Trail as La Jolla Trail. La Jolla is the extended trail to La Jolla Spring, following an unpaved road from the lower Ballard Camp for a half mile to a tiny spring. The fire road to La Jolla Spring returns south for 1.7 miles to Figueroa Road—0.8 mile west of the ranger station and 1.2 miles west of the initial trailhead to Ballard Camp.

🚶	MILESTONES	
►1	0.0	Trail starts opposite the turnoff to Tunnel Road.
►2	0.2	Pass over a seasonal stream.
►3	0.8	Stop at a lookout point above the Santa Ynez Valley.
►4	1.5	The trail levels out at the canyon floor.
►5	1.7	The first campsite is located along the creek.
►6	2.3	The second campsite marks the turnaround.

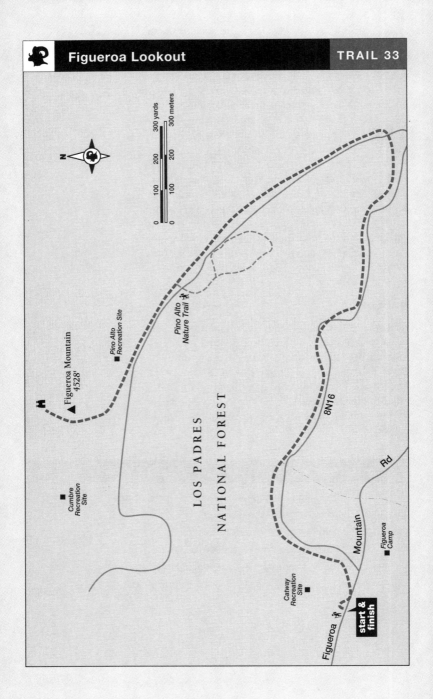

300 yards

300 meters

N

300

300

200

200

100

100

0

0

Pino Alto
Nature Trail

Figueroa Mountain
4528'

Pino Alto
Recreation Site

8N16

LOS PADRES

NATIONAL FOREST

Cumbre
Recreation
Site

Mountain

Rd

Figueroa
Camp

Catway
Recreation
Site

Figueroa

start &
finish

Figueroa Lookout

The pinnacle of the Figueroa Mountain Recreation Area, this fire-road trail is a fun trip by foot, mountain bike, or horseback. It stops at the Pino Alto Nature Trail and then climbs up to the Figueroa Lookout, which offers panoramic views of the San Rafael Wilderness. The short Pino Alto loop is an easy boardwalk trail that is ideal for hikers of all ages. Bikes and horses are not allowed on the boardwalk portion of the trail. Both the lookout and Pino Alto walk offer picnic tables that gaze out over some of the best views the region has to offer.

Best Time

This road, which rises to 4,528 feet, is lined with tall pines and firs that offer shade in the summer. The mountaintop can get very cold in the winter, so fall, spring, and summer hikes are best bets.

Finding the Trail

From Santa Barbara, take Hwy. 101 to the Hwy. 154/Cachuma Lake exit. Head northwest on Hwy. 154/San Marcos Pass, past the Cachuma Recreation Area. When you reach the small town of Los Olivos, make a right on Figueroa Mountain Road and follow the winding road for 13 miles. The trail—marked as Forest Road 8N16 on most maps—is 1.0 mile past the Figueroa ranger station, just after a right-hand turnoff to Tunnel Road and a left-hand turnoff to Forest Road 8N02. Park in the dirt turnoff on the side of the road without blocking access on either road. An Adventure Pass is required.

TRAIL USE
Hike, Run, Bike, Horse
LENGTH
4.45 miles, 3.0 hours
VERTICAL FEET
±868
DIFFICULTY
– 1 2 3 4 **5** +
TRAIL TYPE
Out & Back
SURFACE TYPE
Dirt

FEATURES
Permit Required
Steep
Mountain
Stream
Fall Color
Birds
Wildflowers
Wildlife
Great Views
Camping

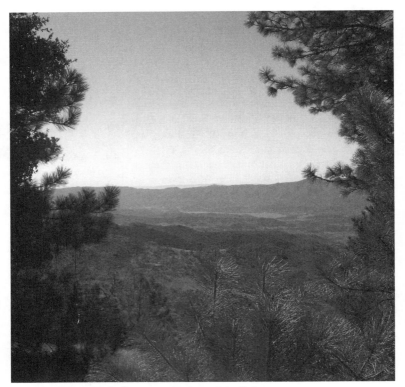

Pino Alto Nature Trail *offers views extending to Lake Cachuma.*

Trail Description

The trail has a fun downhill on the return trip, but at the start offers a challenging climb—starting at 3,600 feet and **rising 1,000 feet in 2.5 miles**. The path starts at the main road ►1 and heads north before circling to the east past the Catway Recreation Site at 0.2 mile. The road crosses a seasonal stream at 0.3 mile ►2 and reaches the 4,000-foot mark at 0.8 mile, where it makes a sharp turn to the north again at just under 1.0 mile.

The Pino Alto Nature Trail is to the left at 1.6 miles. ►3 This fun, short, handicapped-accessible

 Steep

 Handicap Access

hike, located at an elevation of 4,330 feet, is not open to bikes or horses; it is a quick 0.55-mile loop that can be completed in less than a half hour. At the trailhead, you'll see a kiosk offering interpretive trail guides. Stay left from the onset and follow the boardwalk in a clockwise fashion. Follow the boardwalk for 0.25 mile to a clearing among the big-cone Douglas firs, where you'll get a breathtaking view of Lake Cachuma below. The loop can be completed in another 0.25 mile.

The Pino Alto Nature Trail is a self-guided loop trail that gives hikers a sense of the flora and fauna of Figueroa Mountain.

After exiting the nature trail, return to the fire road and stay right at the fork. The left fork heads to the Cumbre parking area, while the Figueroa Lookout can be accessed via the right fork in 0.35 mile. ▶4 The climb is complete at 2.5 miles, including the nature trail loop, and tops out at 4,528 feet. There are picnic tables and restrooms at the summit, which allow those who have conquered it to enjoy the view before retreating back down the way they came. Stay to your right on the way back and remain cautious of oncoming traffic. The return trip to the parking area ▶5 is just under 2.0 miles when you bypass the nature trail.

More to Do at Figueroa Mountain

OPTIONS

Figueroa Mountain might be in the Los Padres National Forest, but with all of those big-cone Douglas fir, ponderosa, and Jeffery pines at the upper elevations, this recreation area has a Sierra Nevada feel to it.

Year-round creeks in the Figueroa include Fir Canyon, Davy Brown, and Manzana.

Along with the hike-in Ballard camps, there are four family campgrounds in this recreation area as well, including Figueroa (33 sites), Davy Brown (13), Nira (12), and Cachuma (7). You can drive to the four campgrounds, although large trailers aren't recommended, as many of the access roads are no longer paved. For more information, contact the Santa Lucia Ranger District at (805) 925-9538.

Notice

Don't be scared off by the steep elevation gain and mileage of this hike. If you're not up to covering 4.45 miles and an 868-foot elevation gain, you can always drive to the nature trail or the lookout point. Keep in mind the road is not paved, and long trailers are not recommended, although the dirt fire road is usually in pretty good shape once the late spring and summer seasons roll around.

🚶	MILESTONES	
▶1	0.00	Follow Forest Road 8N16, accessible from the turnout on Figueroa Mountain Road.
▶2	0.30	The road passes a seasonal stream as it climbs to the lookout area.
▶3	1.60	The Pino Alto Nature Trail is on the left-hand side.
▶4	2.15	After completing the nature trail loop, return to 8N16 and stay right toward the lookout.
▶5	4.50	Return to the parking area via 8N16.

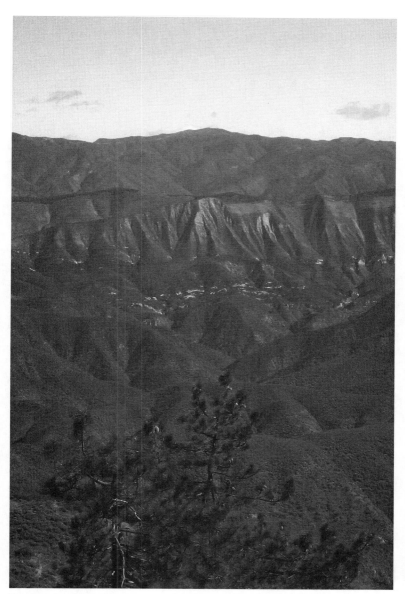

Figueroa Lookout *offers views out to the wilderness charred by the 2007 Zaca Fire.*

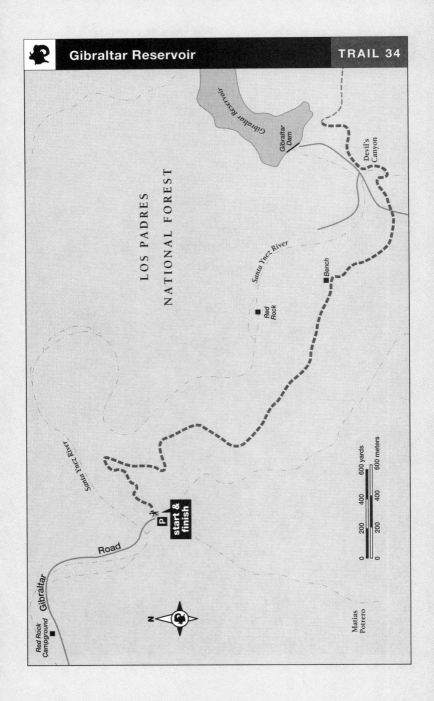

LOS PADRES NATIONAL FOREST

Gibraltar Reservoir

Gibraltar Dam

Devil's Canyon

Santa Ynez River

Bench

Red Rock

Santa Ynez River

start & finish

P

Road

Gibraltar

Red Rock Campground

Matias Potrero

N

0   200   400   600 yards
0   200   400   600 meters

Gibraltar Reservoir

Many people have never even heard of Gibraltar Dam, let alone hiked or ridden there. It was constructed from 1914 to 1920 on the Santa Ynez River, creating the basin for Gibraltar Reservoir, which now provides water for Santa Barbara. The reservoir is accessible via two trails.

The popular Red Rock Trail is a single track that crosses the Santa Ynez River several times and spits out at a popular swimming hole on the river. The second way there is a dirt access road to the dam, which is used a lot less and provides a challenging climb and a fun downhill for mountain bikers and trail runners hoping to avoid the crowds that flock to the Santa Ynez Recreation Area.

Best Time

Because the road to the trailhead and the trail itself can get flooded during the rainy season, the trail is at its best in the summer and fall. The first half of the hike offers little shade, and no drinking water is available along the way, so be sure to pack plenty when hiking in the afternoon.

Finding the Trail

From Hwy. 101 in northern Santa Barbara, take Hwy. 154 west toward Lake Cachuma and turn right on Paradise Road. Follow Paradise Road for 10 miles to the first river crossing. After crossing the river, hang a right and follow Forest Road 5N18 along the river to the Red Rock day-use area. Because the road crosses through the river a couple of times, small

TRAIL USE
Hike, Run, Bike, Horse
LENGTH
6.0 miles, 3.0 hours
VERTICAL FEET
±425
DIFFICULTY
– 1 2 3 4 **5** +
TRAIL TYPE
Out & Back
SURFACE TYPE
Dirt

FEATURES
Permit Required
Dogs Allowed
Canyon
Mountain
Stream
Lake
Birds
Wildflowers

FACILITIES
Restrooms
Picnic Tables
Campground

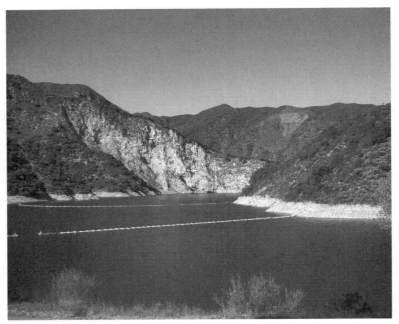

The Gibraltar Reservoir *can be reached only by foot or by bike.*

cars are not recommended. The gated trailhead to the dirt fire road is just past the campground on the far end of the parking lot. An Adventure Pass, available at the Paradise Road ranger station and sometimes at the kiosk before the first river crossing, is required to park in this portion of the Los Padres National Forest.

Trail Description

Pass the gate at the trailhead ▶1 and begin the quick climb via the old access road to the dam. Like you will before many hikes that start with a **rigorous climb**, you may find a 5- to 10-minute warm-up beforehand is a good idea to help prevent strains on the way up. The dirt road takes you high above the

⬛ **Steep**

crowds, which can be heard screaming in the pools below. At 0.87 mile, these turquoise pools ▶2 can be seen down at the base of Red Rock.

When the trail hits the 1.0-mile mark, it has already climbed about 400 feet. ▶3 After a short descent, the trail continues a slow, steady climb over the second mile. Remember to enjoy the sights and sounds on the trail instead of focusing only on the grueling climb itself. The dam can be seen after 1.9 miles. You'll find a strategically located bench at the 2.0-mile mark, ▶4 at an elevation of 1,625 feet. Remember this bench, as it will be your best friend on the return trip. The next mile is nearly all downhill, until the trail finally meets up with the dam and presents another quick climb to the reservoir.

The trail passes the trailhead to Devil's Canyon at 2.5 miles and reaches the **Santa Ynez River** at 2.65 miles, ▶5 dropping down to an elevation of

River

Santa Ynez River Fishing

NOTES

The river can be a fun retreat for Central Coast anglers, once they get a handle on the fishing regulations. While the river and its tributaries downstream from Lake Cachuma's Bradbury Dam are closed to fishing, the stretch above, from Lake Cachuma to Gibraltar Dam, is open to year-round fishing with a bag limit of two trout. The river is usually stocked near the ranger station and campgrounds along Forest Road 5N18 during the general trout season. Check current Department of Fishing and Game regulations, as rules can change in midseason. Because this river is home to wild rainbow trout, anglers are encouraged to use barbless hooks and practice catch and release.

Small panther martins and rooster tails are always solid spin-fishing options on inland streams or rivers like the Santa Ynez. Fly-anglers fall back on tiny dry flies and terrestrials during afternoon hatches in the summer and fall months. Nymphs fished in deeper water will work for trout in the mornings, while streamers are often used for smallmouth bass and panfish near the reservoir.

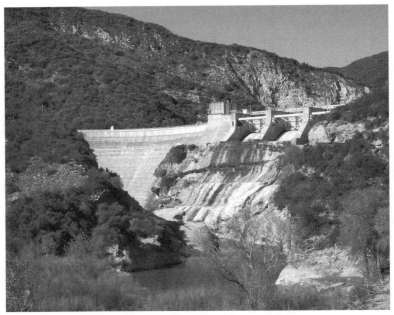

Gibraltar Reservoir *was formed by the damming of Santa Ynez River.*

1,200 feet. This stretch of the river up to the dam has been closed to the public; in fact, much of the dam area and the reservoir are off-limits.

To get the best glimpse of the reservoir, continue up the trail past the dam to a driveway at 3.0 miles, ►6 which leads to the water station. Respect the private property markers at the station, but make sure to pause and soak in all the sights the bright blue reservoir has to offer. This is a good turnaround spot, keeping in mind the trail closes at sunset. The trail does continue around the perimeter of the **lake** and offers views of an old mercury mine, a walk that will tack another 3.0 miles onto the trip. Return the way you came, making sure to take a break at the strategically placed bench before cruising the final 2.0 miles back to the car.

 Lake

Notice

The Devil's Canyon Trail, located 2.5 miles into the Gibraltar Reservoir hike, is an easy-to-follow single track that traces a small feeder creek for 5.0-plus miles one way.

The trails in this portion of the Los Padres National Forest close at sunset. Hikers are encouraged to leave ample time to return to their cars and drive to the park's main entrance at the first river crossing.

	MILESTONES	
►1	0.00	Pass the gate and begin the quick climb along the ridgeline.
►2	0.87	Red Rock is visible to the left beyond the Santa Ynez River swimming holes.
►3	1.00	The trail has already climbed more than 400 feet and begins to flatten out.
►4	2.00	A bench marks an ideal resting spot before the descent to the dam area.
►5	2.65	The trail passes the Santa Ynez River and continues up to the water station.
►6	3.00	The water station marks the turnaround; return the way you came.

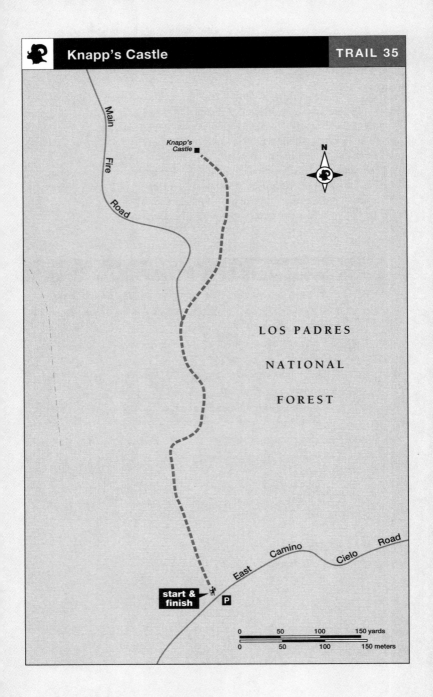

Knapp's Castle

TRAIL 35

Knapp's Castle

N

LOS PADRES

NATIONAL

FOREST

Main Fire Road

East Camino Cielo Road

start & finish

P

| 0 | 50 | 100 | 150 yards |
| 0 | 50 | 100 | 150 meters |

Knapp's Castle

Knapp's Castle isn't exactly a palace anymore, but the milelong hike to its ruins is a fun getaway for hiking couples looking for a nice place to picnic and overlook the Santa Ynez River valley. Brick arches, entryways, and chimneys are all that remain of George Knapp's once-magnificent mountain lodge— a seven-building sandstone masterpiece built in 1916 that was destroyed by a wildfire in 1940.

Best Time

The hike to "the Castle" follows a public fire road for the most part, which makes the trail accessible most of the year. The trail can get rather warm during afternoons in the summer months, so bring water. Mornings and midweek hikes bring the most solitude.

Finding the Trail

From Hwy. 101 in Santa Barbara take the Hwy. 154 exit and follow the highway north toward Lake Cachuma for 8.0 miles. Take a right on East Camino Cielo Road, following the winding two-lane road for 3.0 miles to the dirt turnout across from the trailhead. An Adventure Pass is required. There are no facilities or water in the immediate vicinity of the trail.

Trail Description

The trail starts out at above 3,000 feet ►1 and slowly drops to 2,900 feet, where the ruins are located. The

TRAIL USE
Hike, Run, Bike
LENGTH
1.0 mile, 0.5 hour
VERTICAL FEET
± 802
DIFFICULTY
− **1** 2 3 4 5 +
TRAIL TYPE
Out & Back
SURFACE TYPE
Dirt

FEATURES
Permit Required
Child Friendly
Canyon
Lake
Fall Color
Birds
Wildflowers
Wildlife
Great Views
Photo Opportunity
Historic

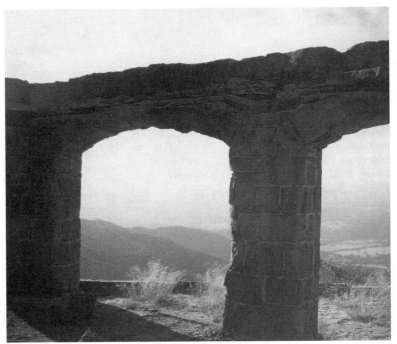

The Santa Ynez River Valley *as seen through the remains of Knapp's Castle*

🚴 **Biking**

🏠 **Historic Interest**

🔭 **Great Views**

fire road continues all the way down to the Santa Ynez River valley and is a popular downhill and return climb for **mountain bikers**. Within the first 0.16 miles of the trail, you will be able to spot the castle's remains, to the northeast. ▶2 At 0.27 mile, the road veers to the left and the trail to the ruins branches off to the right. Head right on the trail past the gate toward the castle. ▶3 The first remnants of **Knapp's Castle** can be seen at 0.41 mile. ▶4. Hike past the rest of the chimneys and arches to where the old balcony once stood, overlooking the valley and Lake Cachuma at 0.5 mile. From here you can see why Knapp chose this spot to build his castle. What a **view**, and a great place to picnic, rest, observe

Painted Cave

Chumash Painted Cave State Historic Park, just south of Knapp's Castle along Hwy. 154, is one of California's smallest state parks. But it packs a historical punch as home to a sandstone cave that houses ancient religious drawings by Chumash Native Americans; some of the red, black, and white images date back to the 1600s.

The park is open from dawn until dusk, with the best views of the cave coming during the middle of the day when the sun is overhead. The cave is protected by a locked iron gate, but if you bring a flashlight, you can see all the images the cave has to offer. On a bright day, you'll be able see religious images and paintings of figures that likely represent the anglers who once patrolled the waters off the Santa Barbara coast. The images were painted or drawn in charcoal, red ochre, and light-colored paints made from powdered shells. Some believe the black circle on the right side of the wall depicts a solar eclipse that occurred in 1677. The cave is believed to have been a regular retreat for Chumash shamans, or priests, who came here seeking power or spiritual strength. There is a short but worthwhile trail that winds around to the top of the cave and offers fine views of the Santa Barbara coastline.

To reach the park, take Hwy. 154, which is about 5.5 miles north of Santa Barbara, to Painted Caves Road and pull over in the dirt turnout at 2.2 miles. Use caution when driving or crossing the narrow, winding road, which is not recommended for trailers or RVs.

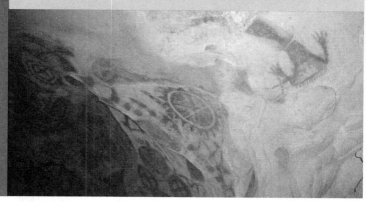

Painted Cave *is one of the smallest state parks.*

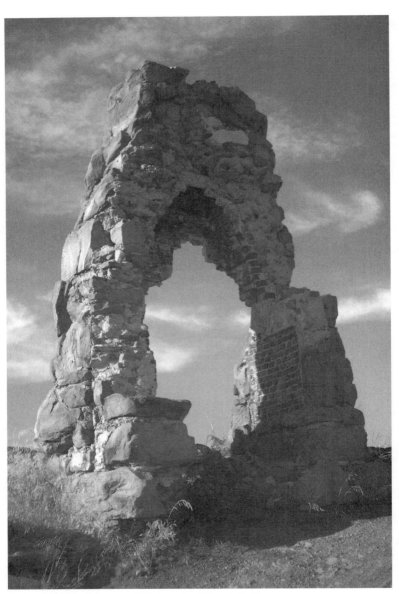

Arches and fireplaces *are all that remain of Knapp's Castle.*

wildlife, take in a sunset, or just to take a breather during your drive through the San Marcos Pass.

When you've seen everything the trail has to offer, trace your steps through the ruins and follow the trail and fire road ►5 back to the parking area.

Notice

Keep in mind that portions of the trail run through private property. The owners have kept the portion of the trail running from the fire road to the ruins open to the public, so stay on trail and respect the ruins and surrounding area.

🚶	MILESTONES	
►1	0.00	The trail is one of few covered in this book that descends from the start, and drops down about 100 feet.
►2	0.16	The ruins can be seen off to the northeast.
►3	0.27	The trail to the ruins branches off the main fire road to the right.
►4	0.40	Reach the ruins at 0.4 mile.
►5	0.50	After exploring the ruins, return the way you came.

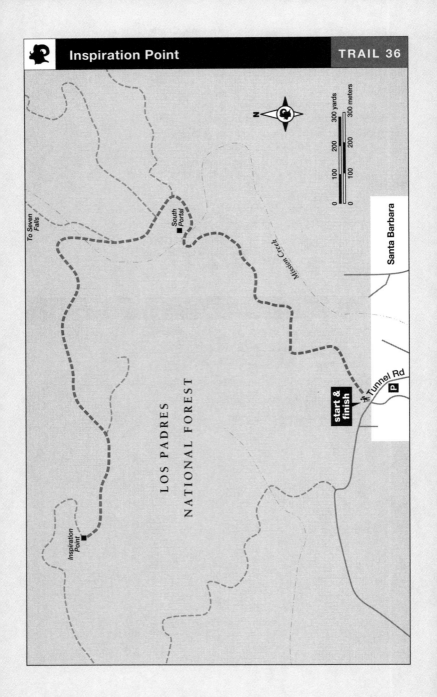

N

300 yards
300 meters
200
200
100
100
0
0

Santa Barbara

To Seven Falls

South Portal

Mission Creek

LOS PADRES NATIONAL FOREST

Tunnel Rd

P

start & finish

Inspiration Point

Inspiration Point

The name says it all. The views from Santa Barbara's Inspiration Point *are* inspirational, to say the least. And making the hike all the way to the overlook point is quite exhilarating. The trail starts on a service road and then winds through shady creekside chaparral to an undefined summit. While there is no clear-cut zenith to this hike, you'll know you've reached the top when you see the views of the city, ocean, and the islands across the channel.

TRAIL USE
Hike, Run, Bike
LENGTH
3.6 miles, 1.5 hours
VERTICAL FEET
±1100
DIFFICULTY
– 1 2 **3** 4 5 +
TRAIL TYPE
Out & Back
SURFACE TYPE
Mixed

FEATURES
Dogs Allowed
Canyon
Stream
Waterfall
Fall Color
Birds
Great Views
Photo Opportunity

Best Time

Because the best part about this trail is the view, this hike is at its best on sunny days. On haze-free afternoons, hikers can look out on the Santa Barbara coast and see the Channel Islands off in the distance. This is a very popular hike throughout the year, so morning hikes during the week get the least amount of traffic. The trail is a hot spot for dog walkers in the late afternoon and evening.

Finding the Trail

From Hwy. 101 in Santa Barbara, exit at Mission St. and drive 1.1 miles to the Santa Barbara Mission. Make a left on Laguna St. and drive past the mission for 0.2 mile. Head right on Los Olivos for 0.7 mile until it becomes Mission Canyon Road. At the stop sign, turn right on Foothill Road for less than 0.2 mile and make a left back onto Mission Canyon Road near the fire station. Make one last left on Tunnel Road and follow it for 1.1 miles to the turnout below the iron gate at the trailhead. Park off the road and avoid blocking residential driveways.

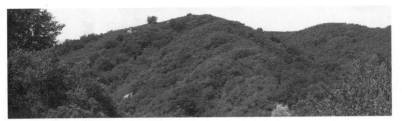

The hike to Inspiration Point is grueling, *but the view from the top is worth it.*

Trail Description

The trail begins at a signed iron gate ▶1 and offers instant views of the Santa Barbara coast. The lower stretches of the trail follow a partially paved road that winds around the canyon and leads to a water station on the creek about 0.6 mile into the hike. Cross the bridge over **Mission Creek,** ▶2 making sure to look down and see the small waterfall that tumbles below.

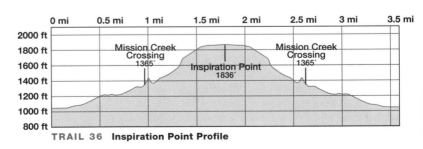

Stream

Continue down the road, which ends at 0.72 mile. Stay left after the road ends ▶3 and follow the signs to the Tunnel and Jesusita trails. At 0.8 mile, the trail splits. Again, stay left and follow the signs to the Tunnel and Jesusita trails. At just under 1.0 mile, the trail runs into the creek again. The first major pool on the creek, a top swimming hole for kids looking to cool off in the summer, is at 1.0 mile. You'll find more pools farther upstream, accessible via the Seven Falls Trail.

TRAIL 36   Inspiration Point Profile

You'll have to do some rock hopping across the creek ►4 to continue on to Inspiration Point. Follow the trail to the left, avoiding the trail that heads right and follows the creek upstream to the falls. At 1.15 miles, you've climbed to the 1,400-foot mark, and the views of the Santa Barbara coast only improve with the climb. As the trail continues, it runs along a small feeder creek that dribbles down to Mission Creek below.

A handful of switchbacks climb the final leg to the summit. The single track hits a crossroad ►5 at 1.6 miles, intersected by an unnamed fire road. Continue straight across the fire road. The overlook is at 1.8 miles, ►6 offering some of the **best views** Santa Barbara has to offer. On the clearest of days, the view spans from Ventura all the way up to San Luis Obispo County. From here, return to the parking lot via the same trail.

 Great Views

Notice

Mountain bikers are encouraged to wear the bells located in a box near the trailhead to alert hikers along their ride.

🚶	**MILESTONES**	
►1	0.0	The trail starts out above the parking area at an iron gate and follows a partially paved service road.
►2	0.6	Cross over the bridge and continue down the road.
►3	0.7	When the road ends, take the single track to the left that leads to the Tunnel and Jesusita trails.
►4	1.0	The trail crosses the creek; take the trail to the left, which ascends to the summit.
►5	1.6	Continue straight on the trail, ignoring a fire road that intersects the trail.
►6	1.8	Check out the overlook and then return the way you came.

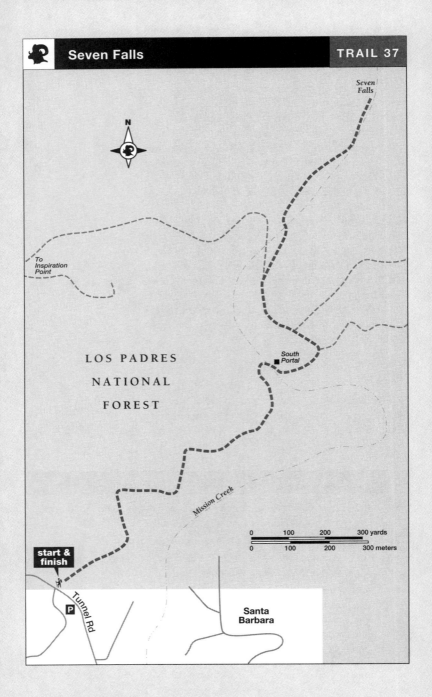

N

Seven
Falls

To
Inspiration
Point

LOS PADRES

NATIONAL

FOREST

South
Portal

Mission Creek

| 0 | 100 | 200 | 300 yards |
| 0 | 100 | 200 | 300 meters |

start &
finish

Tunnel Rd

P

Santa
Barbara

Seven Falls

Many of the directions for this Santa Barbara trail are the same as for Inspiration Point, but some consider Seven Falls a better alternative because it follows a technical single track upstream to a handful of pools filled by bubbling cascades. While the beginning stretches of the two hikes are similar, the trails are two unique stretches that stand on their own. Seven Falls doesn't see as much hiking pressure because it is a smaller, narrower trail, although its pools are popular with swimmers in the summer.

Best Time

While the draw for Inspiration Point is the view, the creek is the draw for the Seven Falls hike. If it's foggy or hazy along the coast, opt for Seven Falls, which is at its highest flows shortly after the rainy season and in the early summer. Hiking during the week is always a good idea on the trails around Mission Creek, as they can get bombarded by walkers, runners, and mountain bikers on the weekends.

Finding the Trail

From Hwy. 101 in Santa Barbara, exit at Mission St. and drive 1.1 miles to the Santa Barbara Mission. Make a left on Laguna St. and drive past the mission for 0.2 mile. Head right on Los Olivos for 0.7 mile until it becomes Mission Canyon Road. At the stop sign, turn right on Foothill Road for less than 0.2 mile and make a left back onto Mission Canyon Road near the fire station. Make one last left on Tunnel Road and follow it for 1.1 miles to the

TRAIL USE
Hike, Run
LENGTH
2.6 miles, 1.5 hours
VERTICAL FEET
±845
DIFFICULTY
– 1 2 3 **4** 5 +
TRAIL TYPE
Out & Back
SURFACE TYPE
Mixed

FEATURES
Dogs Allowed
Canyon
Stream
Waterfall
Fall Color
Birds
Great Views
Photo Opportunity

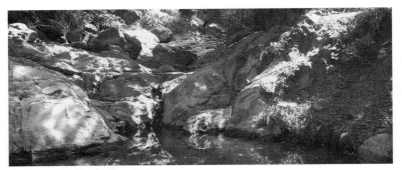

One of the lower pools *on Mission Creek*

turnout below the iron gate at the trailhead. Park off the road and avoid blocking residential driveways.

Trail Description

The trail begins at a signed iron gate ►1 and offers instant views of the Santa Barbara coast. The lower stretches of the trail follow a partially paved road that winds around the canyon and leads to a water station on the creek at 0.6 mile. Cross the bridge over **Mission Creek**, ►2 stopping briefly to look at the small waterfall below.

Continue down the road, which ends at 0.72 mile. Stay left after the road ends ►3 and follow the signs to the Tunnel and Jesusita trails. At 0.8 mile, the trail splits. Again, stay left, and follow the signs to the Tunnel and Jesusita trails.

At just under a mile, the trail runs into the creek again. The first major pool on the creek is 1.0 mile. This is a favorite spot for kids looking to cool off in the summer. Cross the creek ►4 and follow the trail right upstream to the pools. The trail that veers off to the left heads up to Inspiration Point.

This is where the trail becomes technical, getting narrower as the hike continues to wind through the big boulders that parallel the creek. At 1.10 miles, the trail weaves in and out of chaparral cover ►5,

🏞 **Stream**

forcing hikers to duck and dodge some low-hanging
limbs along the way. This portion of the hike could
be tough for taller hikers but offers some **welcome**
shade during the summertime.

 Cool & Shady

At 1.2 miles, the first pool can be spotted off
to the right side of the trail. This is a good vantage
point for seeing Mission Creek below, which carves
through the mini-gorge and tumbles down from
the mountains that make the backdrop for Santa
Barbara Mission.

The trail descends to the creek and peters out at
1.3 miles, where the seven pools are located. ▶6 The
falls between each pool are most impressive after
a heavy rainy season. This is the turnaround spot:
Those looking for a longer hike can return to the
first creek crossing and continue up to Inspiration
Point, another easy-to-follow, out-and-back trail.

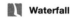 **Waterfall**

Notice

While mountain bikes are allowed on the lower
stretches of this trail, the single track is too technical
for bikes after the first creek crossing at 1.0 mile.

🚶	MILESTONES	
▶1	0.0	The trail starts out above the parking area at an iron gate and follows a partially paved service road.
▶2	0.6	Cross over the bridge and continue down the road.
▶3	0.7	When the road ends, take the single track to the left that leads to the Tunnel and Jesusita trails.
▶4	1.0	The trail crosses the creek; take the trail that parallels the creek upstream.
▶5	1.1	Hike carefully on this technical portion of the trail, winding through boulders and low-handing chaparral.
▶6	1.3	Descend to the turnaround spot at the pools.

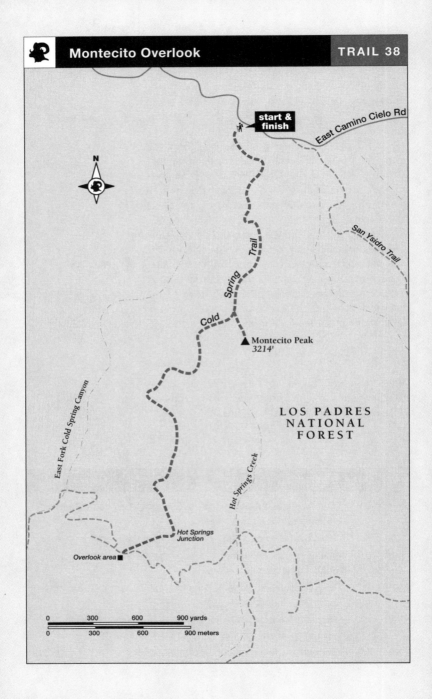

Montecito Overlook · **TRAIL 38**

start & finish

East Camino Cielo Rd

N

San Ysidro Trail

Spring Trail

Cold

▲ Montecito Peak
3214'

East Fork Cold Spring Canyon

LOS PADRES
NATIONAL
FOREST

Hot Springs Creek

Hot Springs Junction

Overlook area ■

| 0 | 300 | 600 | 900 yards |
| 0 | 300 | 600 | 900 meters |

Montecito Overlook

There are many routes to the Montecito Overlook area, but this one is definitely the quickest way to that magnificent vantage point perched 2,500 feet above the Santa Barbara coastline. But while the descent to the lookout via the Cold Spring Trail is quick and relatively painless, the hike back up to the Cold Spring Saddle parking area is no cakewalk. Throw in a side trip to Montecito Peak, and this hike goes from simple to strenuous in a heartbeat. Why do you think there's a logbook for hikers to sign once they've finally reached the peak? Oh yeah, finding the trailhead is no easy task either.

TRAIL USE
Hike, Run, Bike, Horse
LENGTH
3.0 miles, 2.0 hours
VERTICAL FEET
±800
DIFFICULTY
− 1 2 3 **4 5** +
TRAIL TYPE
Out & Back
SURFACE TYPE
Dirt

FEATURES
Permit Required
Dogs Allowed
Mountain
Steep
Stream
Birds
Wildflowers
Wildlife
Great Views
Photo Opportunity
Secluded

Best Time

This is a great springtime hike when the Santa Ynez Mountains are lush green. There are no facilities nearby, so bring water, especially when hiking during the summer months.

Finding the Trail

Getting to the trailhead is half the journey. This particular route starts at the Cold Spring Trail, whose trailhead is located near the Cold Spring Saddle parking area off East Camino Cielo Road. To get there, take the Mission St. exit in Santa Barbara and head north to the mission. Near the mission, make a left on Laguna St., passing the mission and merging onto Los Olivos St. Make the first right and follow the narrow Mountain Dr. for 2.4 miles to Gibraltar Road and make a left. Follow this equally adventurous road into the Santa Ynez Mountains for 6.3

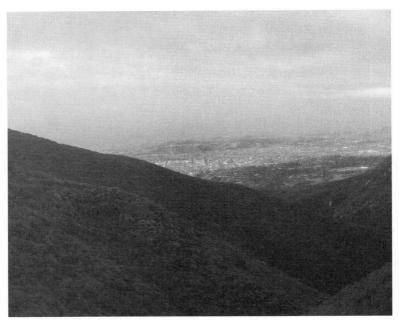

Montecito Peak *towers above Santa Barbara's coastal communities.*

miles before turning right on East Camino Cielo. East Camino Cielo isn't clearly marked, but you'll know you're on the right track if you see a sign pointing the way to Pendola Station. East Camino Cielo also leads to the San Ysidro and Romero trails, among others, so save the directions. Cold Spring Saddle and the trailhead are 3.7 miles east on East Camino Cielo, near the concrete water tank. An Adventure Pass is required for hikes off East Camino Cielo.

Trail Description

Once they finally find the trailhead, hikers are usually eager to get out on the trail. Locate the trailhead sign for the Cold Spring Trail–Mountain Dr. Trail

▶1 and follow the dirt single track south. **Mountain bikers** should pick up bells at the kiosk if they plan on speeding down the hill. (Hikers should note that this route is very popular with downhill riders, who turn the single track into a 4.0-mile point-to-point ride that ends at East Mountain Dr.)

 Biking

Within the first 0.2 mile, you can look down to the Santa Barbara County coast, where even the massive Montecito estates look tiny. ▶2 At 0.6 mile, you'll see Montecito Peak towering above to the southeast. ▶3 The trail hits a rocky section just before the 1.0 mile mark. ▶4 Carefully walk over the crumbly rock, keeping an eye out for a spur on the left-hand side that climbs up to Montecito Peak. The hike to the peak is only 0.5 mile, but it **climbs more than 400 feet along the way**. If you go to the 3,214-foot-high peak, the round-trip adds about a mile to your overall hike.

 Steep

Continue down the Cold Spring Trail for another 0.5 mile, to one of the best lookouts the Santa Barbara coast has to offer. ▶5 This clearing in the mountainside offers tremendous views, from the harbor and pier all the way up to the Gaviota coast. This is a good turnaround spot, as you still have an 800-foot climb over the 1.5 miles back to the car—2.5 miles and 1,200 feet if you want to climb to Montecito Peak.

The side trip to Montecito Peak adds about 1.0 mile to your trip.

Return the way you came, or if you want to go the point-to-point route, continue down the main Cold Spring Trail to East Mountain Dr. Along the way, you'll pass a mini-eucalyptus grove at 1.75 miles, a junction to the Hot Spring Trail at 2.4 miles, and another overlook at 2.6 miles before ending at East Mountain Dr. after about 4.0 miles.

Notice

An Adventure Pass is required to park in many Los Padres National Forest recreation areas, including the East Camino Cielo region. Passes can be purchased at local sporting goods stores and ranger stations.

From the overlook, hikers can see how the stars live. Tucked away among the lower Santa Ynez Mountain foothills, Montecito is considered one of the wealthiest communities in the United States. It has a population of about 10,000 and has been home to such celebrities as Oprah Winfrey and Steven Spielberg.

🚶 MILESTONES

▶1	0.0	Follow the Cold Spring Trail south.
▶2	0.2	Santa Barbara coast is in full view.
▶3	0.6	Locate Montecito Peak to the southeast.
▶4	1.0	A spur on the left leads to the peak.
▶5	1.5	The lookout is located after a handful of switchbacks.

Montecito Peak

The 0.5-mile spur to Montecito Peak is on the south side of the Cold Springs Saddle Trail near the 1.0-mile mark. This steep trail is not regularly maintained and is not recommended for novice hikers. The narrow single track is covered with loose rock, which makes for difficult footing in some places. Be sure to wear solid climbing shoes if you plan on tackling this side trip to the peak.

The path wraps around the peak and reaches the 3,214-foot-high summit from the south, 1.5 miles from the parking area at Cold Springs Saddle. The "peak" is actually a blunt crest where many climbers sit, rest, and soak in the coastal views—writing their thoughts in logbooks stashed in a coffee can atop the mountain.

The views from the peak stretch from the Channel Islands in the south to Goleta in the west. On a clear, sun-soaked day, there might not be a better view in Santa Barbara County. While watching a sunset from the peak is tempting, it's a good idea to make the return trip to the Cold Springs Saddle Trail while there is plenty of daylight remaining.

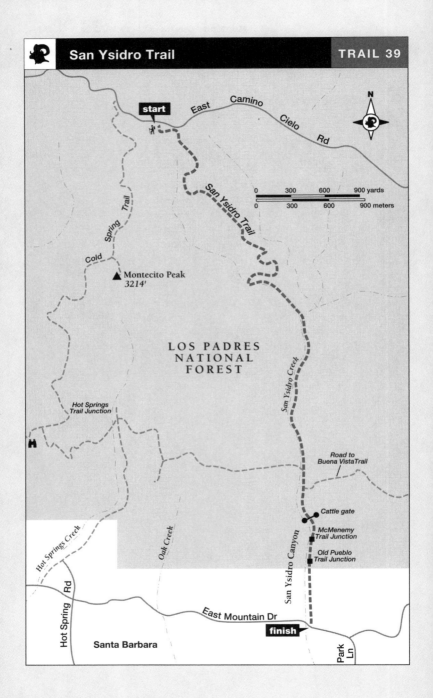

San Ysidro Trail — TRAIL 39

start

East Camino Cielo Rd

N

San Ysidro Trail

Cold Spring Trail

▲ Montecito Peak 3214'

0   300   600   900 yards
0   300   600   900 meters

LOS PADRES NATIONAL FOREST

San Ysidro Creek

Hot Springs Trail Junction

Road to Buena Vista Trail

Cattle gate

McMenemy Trail Junction

Old Pueblo Trail Junction

Hot Springs Creek

Oak Creek

San Ysidro Canyon

Hot Spring Rd

East Mountain Dr

finish

Park Ln

Santa Barbara

San Ysidro Trail

There are few worthwhile point-to-point hikes along the Central Coast and fewer listed in this book. They're a chore to plan and require two vehicles and a hiking companion or somebody who is willing to pick you up at the end of the route and drive back to the trailhead. The San Ysidro Trail, however, with an elevation change of nearly 3,000 feet, is too grueling as an out-and-back hike for most people.

The trail can be a fun, one-way downhill ride for mountain bikers, and a manageable trip down to East Mountain Dr. for intermediate hikers, so the point-to-point route is the most convenient option for those who aren't yet practicing for the Ironman. If solo hikers want to take an out-and-back approach but don't want to log 8.0 miles round trip, the trail description that follows notes a worthwhile turn-around spot at the midway point.

Best Time

This makes a cool winter or springtime hike while the foothills are still lush green. The Santa Ynez Mountains become dry and brown by summer, when morning hikes are best. There are no facilities nearby, so bring water.

Finding the Trail

The trailhead is just past the trailhead to Montecito Peak. To get there, take the Mission St. Exit in Santa Barbara and head north to the mission. Near the mission, make a left on Laguna St., passing the mission and merging onto Los Olivos St. Make the

TRAIL USE
Hike, Run, Bike, Horse
LENGTH
4.0 miles, 2.0 hours
VERTICAL FEET
-2984
DIFFICULTY
- 1 2 3 4 **5** +
TRAIL TYPE
Point-to-Point
SURFACE TYPE
Dirt

FEATURES
Permit Required
Dogs Allowed
Canyon
Mountain
Steep
Stream
Waterfall
Birds
Wildflowers
Wildlife
Great Views
Photo Opportunity

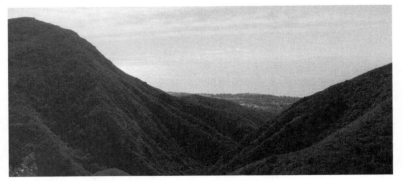

The view from a lookout point *along the San Ysidro Trail*

first right and follow the narrow Mountain Dr. for 2.4 miles to Gibraltar Road and make a left. Follow this equally adventurous road into the Santa Ynez Mountains for 6.3 miles before turning right on East Camino Cielo. East Camino Cielo isn't clearly marked, but you'll know you're on the right track if you see a sign pointing you to Pendola Station. The trailhead is located 0.4 mile east on East Camino Cielo on the right-hand side. An Adventure Pass is required for hikes off East Camino Cielo. This point-to-point hike ends at East Mountain Dr. between San Ysidro Lane and Via Mañana.

Trail Description

 Biking

 Steep

 Great Views

The trail starts at 3,474 feet and follows San Ysidro Creek south ►1 to Santa Barbara. Mountain bike bells to alert hikers of **downhill riders** can be picked up at the trailhead.

The dirt single track starts downhill from the onset, dipping in and out of the shade of San Ysidro Canyon and looking west to Montecito Peak at 0.3 mile. **Panoramic views** of the Santa Barbara coast begin at 0.75 mile. The best unobstructed views of the coast are at the clearing at 1.5 miles, at an elevation of 2,285 feet. This is a good turnaround for

novice out-and-back hikers who want to return to
the parking area at East Cielo. ▶2

Like its sister trail, the Cold Spring Trail, San
Ysidro is a smooth ride on the way down and a grind
on the way back up. Those who want to continue
down to East Mountain Dr. should proceed south on
the main trail, which reaches the 2,000-foot mark
after 2.0 miles. ▶3

You'll know you're on the right track when the
trail crosses the **creek** at 2.4 miles. A spur heads to
the creek again at 2.7 miles, where a waterfall is visible when the flows are high after the rainy season.
▶4 The trail passes junctions to at least three other
trails over the final 2.0 miles. If you continue hiking
south, you'll stay on course. The path intersects the
Buena Vista Trail at around 3.3 miles ▶5 and runs
past an old gate at 3.5 miles.

Two unmarked spurs branch off the main
trail over the final 0.25 mile. Stay straight to East
Mountain Dr., ▶6 which you'll reach at around 4.0
miles at a final elevation of 490 feet.

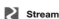 **Stream**

The San Ysidro Trail
is a popular, one-way
downhill mountain
bike trail that spits out
at East Mountain Dr.

Notice

Contact the Santa Barbara Ranger District at (805)
967-3481 for trail conditions and camping information for this portion of the Los Padres National
Forest.

🚶	**MILESTONES**	
▶1	0.0	Follow the creekside trail south.
▶2	1.5	A clearing offers views of the coast.
▶3	2.0	The trail hits the 2,000-foot mark.
▶4	2.4	Reach a creek crossing shortly before a waterfall.
▶5	3.3	Junction with Buena Vista Trail.
▶6	4.0	Trail ends at East Mountain Dr.

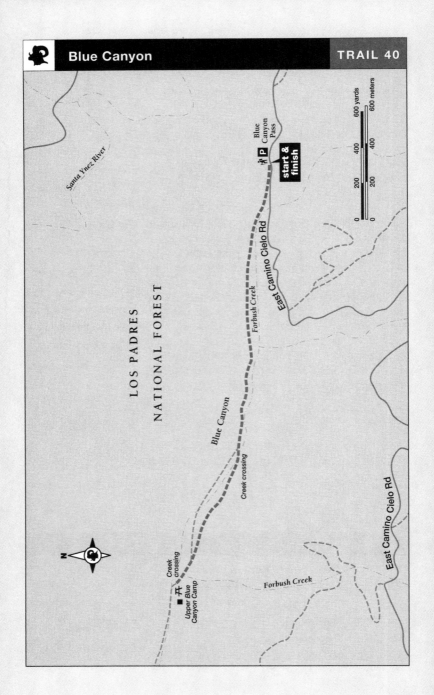

Blue Canyon   TRAIL 40

Blue Canyon

Named after the bluish serpentine that lines the canyon, the Blue Canyon Trail runs alongside Forbush Creek to a handful of oak and sycamore groves that double as camping sites. This particular trail entry ends at Upper Blue Canyon Camp, which is in a creekside grove and is a good stopping place for lunch on a wooden picnic table. The trail continues past here to Cottam and Forbush camps but is narrow and can become overgrown with vegetation and poison oak after the first couple of miles.

TRAIL USE
Hike, Run, Bike
LENGTH
3.2 miles, 1.5 hours
VERTICAL FEET
± 257
DIFFICULTY
– 1 2 **3** 4 5 +
TRAIL TYPE
Out & Back
SURFACE TYPE
Dirt

FEATURES
Permit Required
Child Friendly
Dogs Allowed
Canyon
Stream
Birds
Wildflowers
Camping
Secluded
Geologic

FACILITIES
Picnic Table

Best Time

Because this trail does not receive a lot of pressure in the winter and early spring, the path isn't always clear until late spring and summer. There are no facilities nearby, so bring water or a water filter on summer hikes.

Finding the Trail

Following the same route that takes you to the Montecito Peak and San Ysidro trailheads: Take the Mission St. exit in Santa Barbara and head north to the mission. Near the mission, make a left on Laguna St., passing the mission and merging onto Los Olivos St.

Make the first right and follow the narrow Mountain Dr. for 2.4 miles to Gibraltar Road and make a left. Follow the road into the Santa Ynez Mountains for 6.3 miles before turning right on East Camino Cielo. East Camino Cielo isn't clearly marked, but you'll know you're on the right track

Wearing long sleeves and pants in the spring could help you avoid contacting poison oak on streamside hikes like the Blue Canyon Trail.

if you see a sign pointing you to Pendola Station. Follow East Camino Cielo for 7.0 miles to the Romero Saddle area, where the paved road becomes dirt road. Take the fire road, which is not recommended for small cars, for another 4.0 miles to the trailhead, which is on the north side of the road just after the bridge. A brown forest trail marker marks the trailhead.

Trail Description

The trail starts alongside the road and follows Forbush Creek ▶1 downstream to the west, dropping down through Blue Canyon; the early portions of the dirt single track can get rocky.

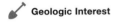 **Geologic Interest**

You'll pass a unique set of **red and yellow sandstone outcroppings** at 0.4 mile. ▶2 A shady grove and spring are around the bend, followed by another batch of sandstone outcroppings at 0.7 mile. This second set has been eroded into statue-like formations along the path.

Stream

From here, the trail drops down to a cliff that overlooks the **creek**, which connects with the larger Santa Ynez River via two intermittent feeder creeks. The trail continues to a bunch of sycamore trees shortly before it crosses one of the tiny tributaries at the 1.0-mile mark. ▶3 Watch for poison oak on this

Western Pond Turtle

NOTES

If you hear a splash along the creekside portions of the Blue Canyon Trail, you've probably startled a western pond turtle. The 5- to 8-inch turtle can be identified by the marble pattern on its shell, along with radiating spots on the carapace. The dark olive or brown turtle seems to prefer slow-moving streams like Forbush Creek where it can bask in the sun on large rocks. While the turtle is common in California, where it is a species of concern, it is nearing extinction in Washington.

lush stretch near the creek. The trail passes another batch of sandstone outcroppings at 1.1 miles and a second tributary at 1.3 miles. ▶4 The path is very unstable along the eroded creek's edge, so hike with caution here.

Climb back up, across the creek to the trail, and continue to the camp at 1.5 miles. ▶5 Here at the first campsite, which is known as Upper Blue Canyon Camp, you'll find a picnic table. A spur on the west side of the **camping spot** leads down to the most accessible portion of the creek at 1.6 miles ▶6. This is a popular spot for hikers hoping to cool off before their return trip to the parking area or for campers who came equipped with a filter and water bottle. The path picks up across the creek but isn't passable during portions of the year because of poison oak and overgrown vegetation. Return the way you came.

 Camping

Notice

An Adventure Pass is traditionally required for hikes in the Santa Ynez River area and trailheads off East Camino Cielo.

🚶	**MILESTONES**	
▶1	0.0	Head west; follow creek downstream.
▶2	0.4	Pass first of many rock outcroppings.
▶3	1.0	Cross the small tributary.
▶4	1.3	Carefully cross over another feeder creek.
▶5	1.5	Reach the camp and picnic table.
▶6	1.6	Follow the spur to the creek and the turnaround.

Northern Ventura County–Channel Islands

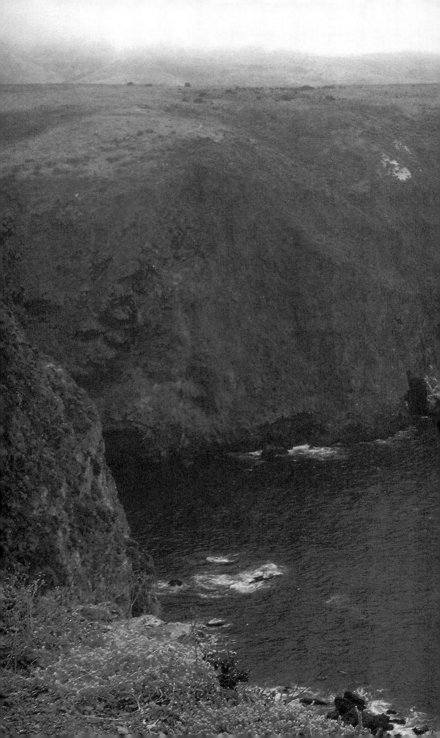

Northern Ventura County– Channel Islands

The hikes in northern Ventura County are reminiscent of the creekside trails that can be found to the north in Santa Barbara, San Luis Obispo, and even Monterey counties. But hop on a boat at Ventura or Channel Islands Harbor, and you'll be miles away from ordinary in no time.

Santa Cruz Island, one of the five islands that make up Channel Islands National Park, is about 20 miles from the Ventura harbor and is the largest and most diverse island in the chain. The 96-square-mile island has two mountain ranges flanked by a central valley and supports more than 1,000 species of plant and animal life. A dozen of those species are found nowhere else in the world. There are more than a dozen hikes on the island, which is why Santa Cruz is the most popular island among outdoor enthusiasts. There are six hikes that begin from near Scorpion Beach, three from Smugglers Cove, and six from Prisoners Harbor.

Visitors should note that much of the west side of the island is owned by the Nature Conservancy and is closed to the public. The boundary between the national park and Nature Conservancy is clearly marked by the fence line between Prisoners Harbor and Valley Anchorage.

Permits and Maps

Island maps and brochures are available at the Channel Islands National Park office at the marina in Ventura. Call (805) 658-5730 or visit www.nps.gov/chis for more information. Camping is available by reservation. You can get maps via the different charter boat outfits that offer trips to the islands, and there is an information kiosk near the pier at Santa Cruz Island where you can purchase maps.

Overleaf and opposite: *Cavern Point offers views of Santa Cruz Island's rugged coast and sea caves.*

Island Packers is the authorized charter company for Channel Islands National Park; the boat drops passengers off at the Scorpion Harbor Pier on east Santa Cruz. Make reservations by calling (805) 642-1393.

Matilija Creek and Santa Paula Canyon are in the Ojai District of the Los Padres National Forest. Los Padres National Forest maps can be viewed at www.fs.fed.us/r5/forestvisitormaps/lospadres or purchased at www.national-foreststore.com. For more information, contact the Los Padres ranger station in Goleta at (805) 968-6640.

Santa Clara River Estuary Natural Preserve is accessible via the campground at McGrath State Beach, where there is a day-use fee. You can get trail information and a park brochure at the entrance kiosk or at the information center.

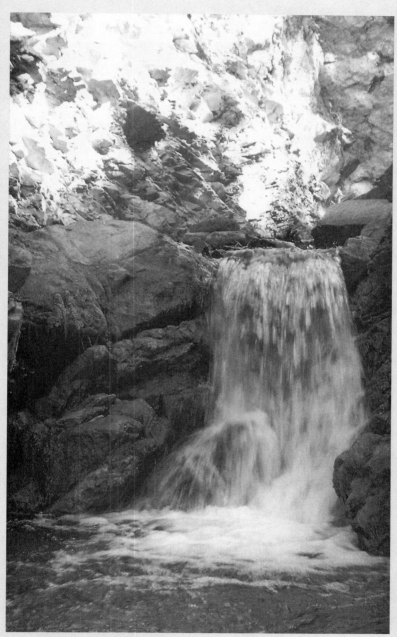

A small cascade *on Santa Paula Creek*

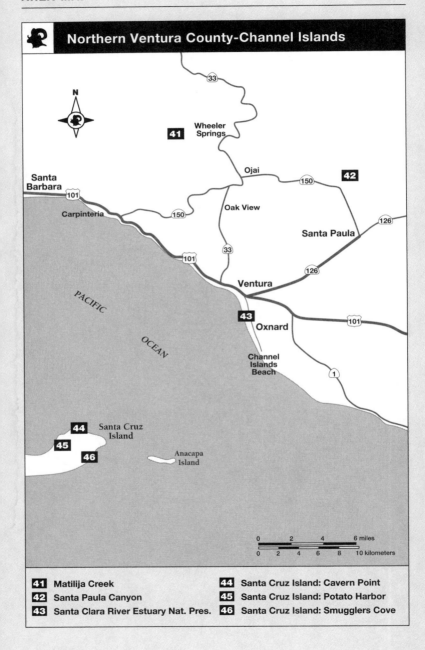

CHAPTER 5

Northern Ventura County-Channel Islands

41 Matilija Creek

42 Santa Paula Canyon

43 Santa Clara River Estuary Nat. Pres.

44 Santa Cruz Island: Cavern Point

45 Santa Cruz Island: Potato Harbor

46 Santa Cruz Island: Smugglers Cove

Northern Ventura County—Channel Islands

TRAIL	Difficulty	Length	Type	USES & ACCESS	TERRAIN	FLORA & FAUNA	OTHER
41	5	13.0	⟋	🚶 🏃 ☑	🔁 ⅡⅠ 🏞 ⛰	🌸 🍁 🐦 🦌	⟋ 👀 ⛺
42	4	6.2	⟋	🚶 🏃	🔁 ⅡⅠ 🏞	🍁 🐦 🦌	⛺ 📷
43	2	1.4	⟋	🚶 🏃 👫 ♿ $	🔁 🏖	🐦 🦌	👀 ⛺
44	2	2.0	↺	🚶 🏃 👫	🏖	🐦	👀 🌲 ↑ 📷
45	2	3.2	⟋	🚶 🏃 👫	🏖	🐦	👀 🌲 ↑ 📷
46	5	7.4	⟋	🚶 🏃 👫	🏖	🐦	👀 🌲 ↑ 📷

USES & ACCESS
- 🚶 Hiking
- 🐎 Horses
- 🏃 Running
- 🚴 Biking
- 👫 Child Friendly
- ♿ Handicap Access
- $ Fee
- ☑ Permit Required
- 🐕 Dogs Allowed

TYPE
- ↺ Loop
- ⟋ Out & Back
- ⟍ Point-to-Point

DIFFICULTY
- 1 2 3 4 5 +
less   more

TERRAIN
- 🔁 River or Stream
- ⅡⅠ Waterfall
- 〰 Lake
- 🏖 Beach
- 🐟 Tide Pools
- 🏞 Canyon
- ⛰ Mountain

FLORA & FAUNA
- 🌸 Wildflowers
- 🍁 Fall Color
- 🐦 Birds
- 🦌 Wildlife

FEATURES
- 🏛 Historic Interest
- ⟋ Geologic Interest
- 👀 Great Views
- ↑ Steep
- ↑ Secluded
- 🌲 Cool and Shady
- ⛺ Camping
- 📷 Photo Opportunity

Northern Ventura–Channel Islands

This backpacking trail hops back and forth along the North Fork of Matilija Creek on its way up to Matilija Camp. Because there are a handful of creek crossings, this can be a challenging hike for backpackers in the spring when flows are high. Pack lightly, and if you're planning an overnight trip, wait until the summer and fall, when flows are more manageable.

It doesn't exactly look like the best place to go for a hike, but once you get past the local college, avocado farms, and oil wells on the lower portions of the canyon, you'll see Santa Paula Creek Canyon is home to a crystal-clear creek and dozens of species of birds and wildlife—not to mention a beautiful waterfall and some fun swimming holes.

While this is a short trail, its nature and beach walk portions crawl through a mishmash of ecosystems, including the ocean, sandy beach, estuary, coastal dunes, saltwater and freshwater marshes, and river and streamside woodlands. This diverse habitat offers some of the best bird-watching opportunities in the region.

Santa Cruz Island: Cavern Point 287

The quickest, easiest hike for those visiting Santa Cruz Island for the day, the Cavern Point hike offers a bird's-eye view of sea caves below, along with a coastal panorama of the mainland. The hike can be completed in less than 45 minutes if you follow the lazy-day loop clockwise to avoid the steepest incline.

TRAIL 44

Hike, Run
2.0 miles, 1.0 hour
Loop
Difficulty: 1 **2** 3 4 5

Santa Cruz Island: Potato Harbor ... 291

Another relatively easy hike, Santa Cruz Island's Potato Harbor Trail leads to another overlook on the north side of Santa Cruz Island. From here, you can peer across to the mainland and down to a protected cove that is shaped like a potato. It's a great perch for wildlife-watchers who want to look down on barking seals and swooping brown pelicans.

TRAIL 45

Hike, Run
3.2 miles, 1.5 hours
Out & Back
Difficulty: 1 **2** 3 4 5

Santa Cruz Island: Smugglers Cove. 295

The hike to Santa Cruz Island's Smugglers Cove is a 7.4-mile trek that is popular with visitors who plan an extended stay. The turquoise cove is hidden from the wind and is a great spot for swimming, body-surfing, sunbathing, or fishing.

TRAIL 46

Hike, Run
7.4 miles, 3.5 hours
Out & Back
Difficulty: 1 2 3 4 **5**

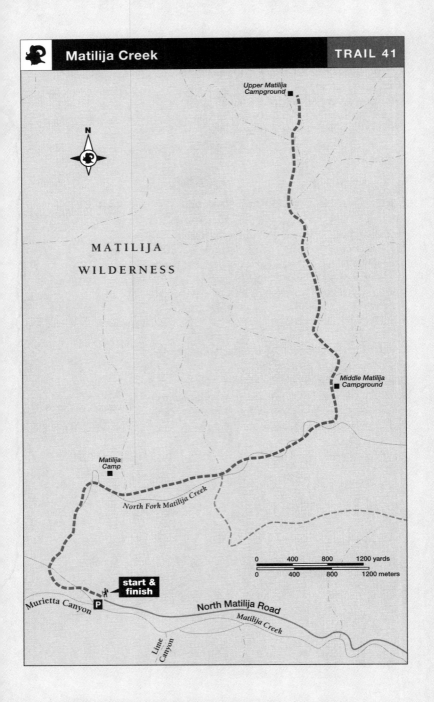

Upper Matilija
Campground ■

N

MATILIJA
WILDERNESS

Middle Matilija
■ Campground

Matilija
Camp ■

North Fork Matilija Creek

| 0 | 400 | 800 | 1200 yards |
| 0 | 400 | 800 | 1200 meters |

start &
finish

P

Murietta Canyon

North Matilija Road

Matilija Creek

*Lime
Canyon*

Matilija Creek

An adventurous summer getaway that includes a handful of camping sites and countless cascades, the Matilija Camp Trail keeps you cool with a number of creek crossings as it weaves its way up the North Fork of Matilija Creek in the Los Padres National Forest. Much of the upper watershed is located within a federally protected wilderness area that is home to endangered steelhead trout and the California condor. The North Fork is one of the few trails that provide access to the remote Matilija Wilderness.

Best Time

Because the flows of the creek are difficult to judge during the winter and spring, this Matilija Creek hike is a lot safer during the summer months when flows are calm. Call the Ojai ranger station at (805) 646-4348 for the latest trail conditions and flow information.

Finding the Trail

From Hwy. 101 in Ventura, take Hwy. 33 exit north toward Ojai. Follow the highway for 17 miles before making a left on Matilija Canyon Road. Follow the road, which begins as South Matilija Road and eventually becomes North Matilija Road on some maps, for 5.0 miles until it dead-ends at a dirt parking area near Matilija Canyon Ranch.

TRAIL USE
Hike, Run

LENGTH
13.0 miles, all day

VERTICAL FEET
±2300

DIFFICULTY
– 1 2 3 4 **5** +

TRAIL TYPE
Out & Back

SURFACE TYPE
Mixed

FEATURES
Permit Required
Canyon
Mountain
Stream
Waterfall
Fall Color
Birds
Wildflowers
Wildlife
Great Views
Camping
Geologic

Trail Description

From the gate, follow the access road through the ranch, remembering to abide by the Forest Service easement and respect private property throughout the lower section of the hike. ►1 The paved road eventually turns to dirt and immediately crosses **Matilija Creek** at 0.1 mile. The path crosses the creek again at the 0.5-mile mark, before the junction to Matilija Camp Trail ►2 and immediately after the crossing on the right-hand side. The trail parallels and sometimes crosses the North Fork of Matilija Creek to the north, where Matilija Camp is located.

You will reach the first camp at 1.4 miles, ►3 set near the river on a flat shaded by oaks and surrounded by boulders. This is a great place to **camp** or, if the site is occupied, to rest briefly. While this camp will be the turnaround point for many hikers, the trail does continue east to three more camps that are worth the trek—especially during the summer months when the first site is usually occupied, thanks to the cool pools rounded out of the sandstone on this narrow stretch of the creek.

After the first campsite, the trail heads east. From here, the trail can become overgrown during the spring and winter months. Just be sure to follow the creek and **canyon** upstream. The trail crosses the creek a handful of times depending on the flows, but runs primarily along the left (northwest) side of the creek. The creek forks at 3.7 miles. The trail turns, north at this point, staying to the west of the fork and running into Middle Matilija Camp around the 4.0-mile mark. ►4

The trail continues for about 2.0 miles to Upper Matilija Camp, which is on the west side of the creek at about 6.0 miles. ►5 Maple Camp is 0.5 mile to the north, some 6.5 miles from the trailhead. ►6 This is the turnaround, as the creek is little more than a trickle at this point. Return the way you came.

Stream

Camping

Canyon

The Matilija Wilderness is home to the endangered southern steelhead and California condor.

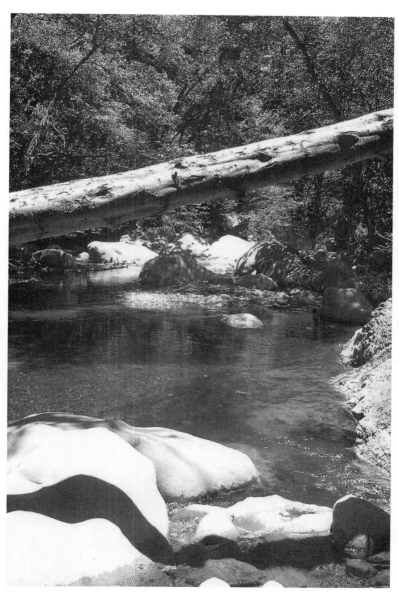

Matilija Creek *is an historic steelhead passageway.*

Ambitious backpackers can continue north for a couple miles to Cherry Creek Camp, which is on the banks of Sespe Creek en route to the northern access point off Hwy. 33.

Notice

Fly-anglers who make multiple creek crossings during a day of fishing often rely on a wading staff to cross from bank to bank. A collapsible wading stick is a good idea for hikers who intend to cross creeks more than once along trails like the Matilija Camp Trail.

Call the Ojai ranger station at (805) 646-4348 for camping information, maps and regulations.

🚶	MILESTONES	
►1	0.0	Start at the gate and follow the road west.
►2	0.5	Road meets Matilija Camp Trail heading to the north.
►3	1.4	Matilija Camp is located along the creek.
►4	4.0	Come to Middle Matilija Camp.
►5	6.0	Trail runs past Upper Matilija Camp.
►6	6.5	Maple Camp marks the turnaround spot.

NOTES

Days Numbered for Matilija Dam

It's only a matter of time before Matilija Creek runs wild again.

In April 2007, the House passed the Water Resources Development Act, authorizing the expenditure of $144.5 million for the removal of Matilija Dam, along with additional restoration projects in the Ventura River watershed. Local conservation groups hope the removal of Matilija Dam—which is about 4.0 miles east of the trailhead to Matilija Camp—will allow the southern steelhead to reach vital backcountry spawning grounds. The trout could enter Matilija Creek via the Ventura River, which runs west to the Pacific. The conservationists argue that the tributary provides some of the best remaining habitat for steelhead. The Matilija was home to thousands of migrating steelhead before the 200-foot-high dam was built for flood control and water storage in 1948. Ventura County officials hope the dam removal project breaks ground by 2012.

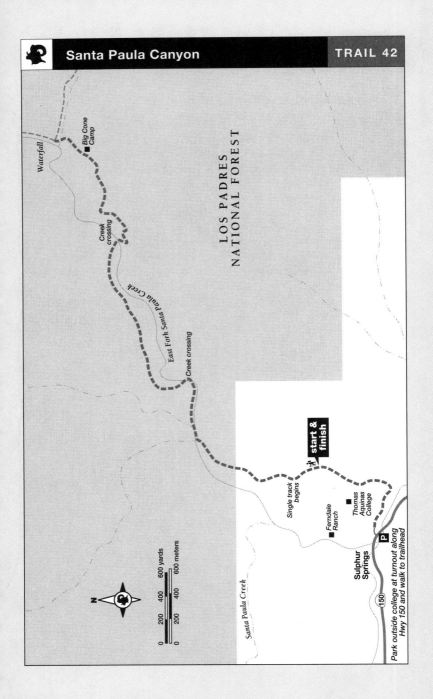

Santa Paula Canyon

TRAIL 42

Waterfall

Big Cone Camp

LOS PADRES NATIONAL FOREST

Creek crossing

East Fork Santa Paula Creek

Creek crossing

start & finish

Single track begins

Thomas Aquinas College

Ferndale Ranch

Sulphur Springs

Santa Paula Creek

Park outside college at turnout along Hwy 150 and walk to trailhead

150

N

0   200   400   600 yards
0   200   400   600 meters

Santa Paula Canyon

Look past the local college, avocado farms, and oil wells that sour the lower portions of the canyon, and you'll see Santa Paula Creek Canyon for what it's supposed to be—an awe-inspiring gorge that's home to a crystal-clear creek, and dozens of species of birds and wildlife.

But like other waterways in the Santa Clara River watershed (Piru and Sespe creeks), the Santa Paula has been subject to the stressors that plague many urban streams—loss of habitat, streambed alteration caused by flood-control structures, and degradation of water quality. Even the trail's giant boulders are plagued by graffiti on the lower stretches of the creek. While conservation efforts are in place to help restore the canyon to a more natural state, the pristine portions of the canyon are up near the falls, more than 3.0 miles upstream from the Hwy. 180 bridge.

Best Time

The creek flows all year long, although it gets swamped by swimmers and campers in the summer months. The best time for a secluded hike is during the week. Bring a sweatshirt if hiking the canyon in the late fall or winter, as much of the trail, blocked by the canyon's steep walls, is in the shade in the early morning and late afternoon.

Finding the Trail

Take Hwy. 126 from Ventura to the town of Santa Paula and take the Hwy. 150 exit toward Ojai.

TRAIL USE
Hike, Run
LENGTH
6.2 miles, 3.0 hours
VERTICAL FEET
±600
DIFFICULTY
– 1 2 3 **4** 5 +
TRAIL TYPE
Out & Back
SURFACE TYPE
Dirt, Gravel

FEATURES
Canyon
Stream
Waterfall
Fall Color
Birds
Wildlife
Photo Opportunity
Camping

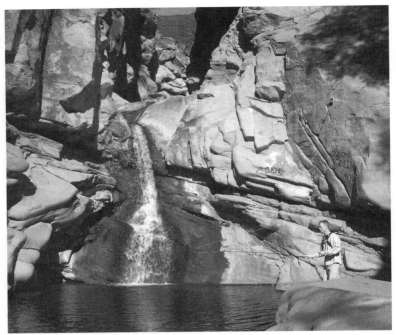

Fly-fishing near the waterfall *at Santa Paula Creek*

Take Hwy. 150 to Thomas Aquinas College and park outside the campus entrance gate. Follow the TRAIL HIKERS signs to the trailhead, which is off the perimeter road that winds counterclockwise around the campus.

Trail Description

The trailhead is in back of Thomas Aquinas College, a four-year Catholic liberal arts school, and it scoots past ranch houses and the thumpity-thump of some rusty oil wells. After the first mile, the eyesores disappear and the trail follows the creek upstream through the towering Topatopa Mountains of the Los Padres National Forest.

The trail, which begins as a dirt road, finally takes shape at 0.6 mile, once the road ends. ►1 Follow the single track to the left around a final set of oils wells and the path will begin to feel like a trail again. Once you reach the **creek**, keep an eye out for brown Forest Service signs marking the trail, which starts upstream along the right side of the creek. Some portions of the trail were flooded and washed away during the winter of 2005, so the brown trail markers are really key in pointing you in the right direction throughout the hike.

Stream

The trail crosses the creek at 1.0 mile ►2 and continues up the left side for a good mile. After the first mile, the trail separates from the creek for a bit and weaves through shrubs and knee-high grasses that are popular with birds and deer. The trail is washed out in a couple of areas near the 2.0-mile mark, which could lead to some boulder hopping along the creek's edge.

Cross the creek at the 2.1-mile mark, where the hard-to-follow trail joins a better-maintained trail that climbs up toward **Big Cone Camp**. ►3 This is the steepest portion of the trail, climbing about 500 feet over the final mile. At 2.9 miles, you can see how far you've come, looking down to the creek below. A shaded Douglas fir grove ►4 is just ahead. Here, before the trail descends back to the creek, you'll find Big Cone Camp and some primitive camping sites.

Camping

Follow the trail through the camp, taking the switchbacks down toward the bottom of the canyon. Once you reach the creek, head left about 50 yards downstream, toward the waterfall, which can be heard crashing around the bend. If you climb upstream immediately after reaching the main fork, you will miss Santa Paula Canyon Falls completely. ►5 The **20-foot waterfall**, at 3.1 miles, ►6 drops down from the East Fork of Santa Paula Creek and meets up with the main creek below as it cascades

Waterfall

into a turquoise pool that is a popular retreat for swimmers. A sandy beach on the right side of the pool, which is the hike's turnaround, is a nice spot for a picnic. The best way back to the parking lot is to return the way you came.

Notice

Backpackers interested in camping in the canyon can stay at Big Cone Camp, located just before the falls. Call the Ojai Ranger District at (805) 646-4348 for availability and permit information.

Horses are allowed on the trail but not recommended now that stretches have been washed out, forcing trail users to cross the creek and boulder hop at many locations.

The best trout fishing on Santa Paula Creek is above the falls and farther up the East Fork and its feeder creeks. Tiny nymphs and dry flies are the norm on this small-water stretch. Small, barbless spinners such as pink panther martins also work for these small, wild trout on the upper stretches.

⋀	MILESTONES	
▶1	0.0	Locate the trailhead on campus and follow the trail signs past the ranch houses and oil wells.
▶2	0.6	The dirt road ends and becomes a single track that heads upstream.
▶3	2.1	Watching for washouts in the trail, cross the creek and follow the maintained trail that ascends to Big Cone Camp.
▶4	2.9	Big Cone Camp and a grove of shaded Douglas fir make for a nice resting point.
▶5	3.0	Follow the switchbacks down to the creek's edge and head downstream for about 50 yards.
▶6	3.1	The waterfall pours down from the East Fork to the main creek, marking the turnaround.

More Santa Paula Canyon Hikes

Serenity may be hard to find in Santa Paula Canyon during the summer months, especially on the weekends. One way to get away from the crowds that flood the creek's swimming holes is to continue hiking past the waterfall.

A secluded alternative to Big Cone Camp is Cross Camp, which is a little less than a mile upstream on the main creek. Hike upstream for another 1.8 miles, and the trail veers right and drops down to Jackson Camp and Jackson Hole. The main trail continues to climb the canyon to Last Chance Camp and hikes high above into the Topatopa Mountains.

Call the Ojai Ranger District at (805) 646-4348 for camping availability and permit information. An Adventure Pass is required for camping in the Los Padres National Forest. The Los Padres Forest Association publishes an Ojai trails guide with a map of Santa Paula Canyon's trails, available at the Ojai ranger station at 1190 East Ojai Dr. in Ojai.

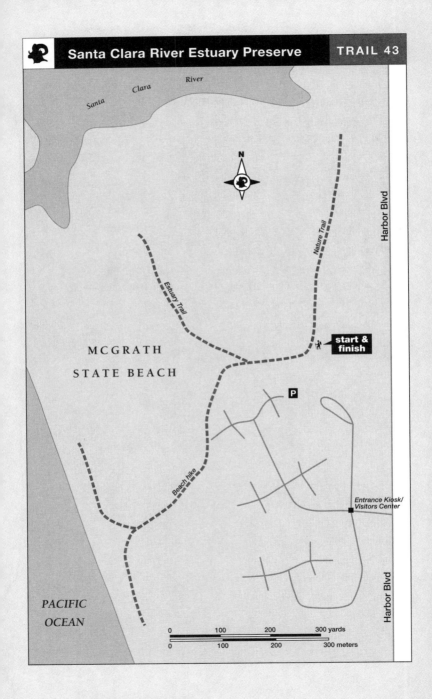

Santa Clara River Estuary Preserve TRAIL 43

Santa Clara River

N

Harbor Blvd

Nature Trail

Estuary Trail

MCGRATH
STATE BEACH

start &
finish

P

Beach hike

Entrance Kiosk/
Visitors Center

PACIFIC
OCEAN

Harbor Blvd

| 0 | 100 | 200 | 300 yards |
| 0 | 100 | 200 | 300 meters |

Santa Clara River Estuary Natural Preserve

The Santa Clara River Estuary Natural Preserve is accessible via a nature trail and multiple spurs leading from the campground at McGrath State Park. Home to hundreds of animal species, the preserve is made up of several unique ecosystems, including the ocean, sandy beach, estuary, coastal dunes, saltwater and freshwater marshes, and river and streamside woodland. The variety of ecosystems provide some of the best bird-watching opportunities this side of Morro Bay.

Best Time

The summer and fall are the best seasons for this hike, as the campground and its trails often become flooded during and beyond the rainy season. But even if the trails on the north side of the campground have been flooded, the west-running spurs to the beach should be open all year and provide access to 2.0 miles of beach.

Finding the Trail

McGrath State Park sits just south of the Ventura Harbor in Oxnard. Take the Seaward Ave. exit off U.S. Hwy. 101, merging onto Harbor Blvd. Follow Harbor south for 4.0 miles, crossing over the Santa Clara River and leaving the Ventura city limits. The entrance to McGrath State Park is on the west side of Harbor Blvd. The trailhead is on the north side of the park, just past the entrance kiosk. A map of the campground and a brochure for the self-guided nature trail is available at the park entrance. There is a day-use fee.

TRAIL USE
Hike, Run
LENGTH
1.4 miles, 1.0 hour
VERTICAL FEET
±52
DIFFICULTY
− 1 **2** 3 4 5 +
TRAIL TYPE
Out & Back
SURFACE TYPE
Dirt

FEATURES
Handicap Access
   (Nature Trail)
Parking Fee
Child Friendly
Stream
Beach
Birds
Wildlife
Great Views
Camping

FACILITIES
Restrooms
Water
Visitors Center

283

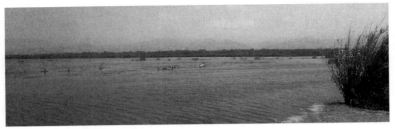

The second leg of the trail *dead-ends at the estuary.*

Trail Description

Find the trailhead to the short nature trail, ▶1 which is on the north side of the campground, just past the entrance kiosk. Follow the nature trail north to the Santa Clara River. This short but informative self-guided hike through the streamside woodland crosses over a boardwalk and is one of the few handicapped-accessible hikes in Ventura County. There are plenty of benches located along the way for a quick rest or picnic beneath the woodland canopy.

The trail dead-ends at the estuary in just 0.15 mile. ▶2 Hiking beyond the turnaround is a bad idea, as the estuary is a mud trap. The end of the nature trail is a fine perch for **bird-watchers**, offering a glimpse of the estuary where the river and saltwater environments mesh. After getting a good look at the shorebirds that frequent the estuary, return to the start of the nature trail at 0.3 mile.

When you reach the earlier trailhead, ▶3 turn right and follow the well-defined but unsigned dirt trail west around the perimeter of the campground. Just before the 0.5-mile mark, a spur heads northwest toward the mouth of the estuary. Follow this spur ▶4 for 0.2 mile to the edge of the river. This is another good vantage point for birding, with views of the dunes and estuary environments, which are popular with the western snowy plover, brown pelican, and northern harrier. The sandy trail is home to reptiles like the legless lizard and small snakes.

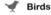 **Birds**

This preserve is composed of several ecosystems—the ocean, sandy beach, estuary, coastal dunes, saltwater and freshwater marshes, and river and streamside woodland.

Return to the main trail, which you'll come to at 0.6 mile, and follow the path west toward the beach. ▶5 The latter portions of the trail, before the short climb over the dunes, can get flooded after heavy rains. If standing water blocks your path, there are additional beach routes to the south, branching off the road that weaves through the campground.

The trail crawls over undulating dunes before spitting out at McGrath State Beach ▶6 at just under 1.0 mile. From here, you can access 2.0 miles of **beach**, which is ideal for wading, surfing, or at the very least, a nice stroll. Return the way you came, following the main path for less than a 0.5 mile back to the day-use parking area.

 Beach

Notice

Call McGrath State Park at (805) 968-1033 for current trail conditions, as the river often floods the campground and nearby trails.

	MILESTONES

▶1	0.00	The nature trail is located near the day-use parking area.
▶2	0.15	Nature trail ends; return to the main trail.
▶3	0.30	Follow the main track west toward beach.
▶4	0.45	Spur leads to the river's edge.
▶5	0.60	Return to main trail; continue west to beach.
▶6	1.00	Trail reaches beach, the turnaround spot.

McGrath State Beach

OPTIONS

McGrath State Beach has more than 170 year-round campsites, but it is usually jam-packed throughout the summer because it is situated smack-dab in the middle of Ventura and Oxnard, near the wharf. With a 2.0-mile stretch of beach, the area is popular with sun bathers, surf anglers, swimmers, surfers, and kayakers.

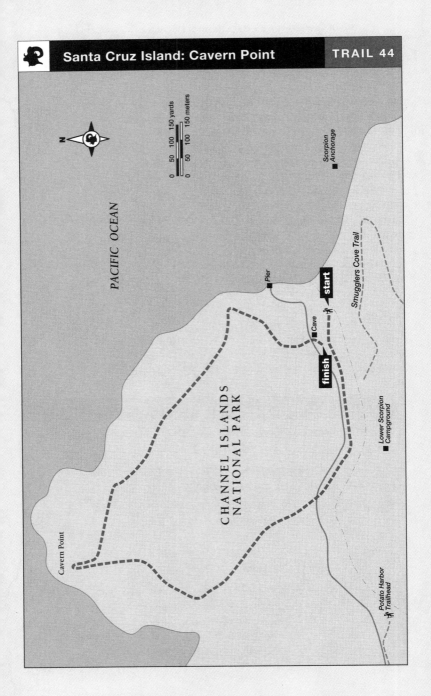

PACIFIC OCEAN

Scorpion
Anchorage

150 yards

150 meters

100

100

50

50

0

0

Pier

Smugglers Cove Trail

start

Cave

finish

CHANNEL ISLANDS
NATIONAL PARK

Lower Scorpion
Campground

Cavern Point

Potato Harbor
Trailhead

Santa Cruz Island: Cavern Point

The Cavern Point Trail is a painless Channel Islands hike perfectly suited for visitors making a day trip to Santa Cruz Island. The trail is defined by its breathtaking views of sea caves below, along with a coastal panorama of the mainland. It can be completed in less than an hour if you follow the lazy-day loop clockwise to avoid the steepest incline.

Best Time

The Cavern Point hike is a good year-round stroll that's best on clear, fog-free days. The island sees warm temperatures in the summer, which makes a picturesque hike at sunrise and sunset that much more appealing.

Finding the Trail

Island Packers is the authorized charter company for Channel Islands National Park. Make reservations by calling (805) 642-1393. The boat leaves out of Channel Islands Harbor in Ventura and drops passengers off at the Scorpion Harbor Pier on east Santa Cruz Island. Take the fire road from the pier past Scorpion Ranch for 0.2 mile to the clearly marked trailhead at the beginning of the first campground.

Trail Description

The trail starts out of the lower Scorpion Campground ►1 and climbs to its highest point at just over 300 feet above sea level. Look for **island foxes** near the campground, where they sometimes can be found searching for food even during daylight hours.

TRAIL USE
Hike, Run
LENGTH
2.0 miles, 1.0 hour
VERTICAL FEET
±300
DIFFICULTY
− 1 **2** 3 4 5 +
TRAIL TYPE
Loop
SURFACE TYPE
Dirt

FEATURES
Child Friendly
Steep
Beach
Birds
Great Views
Photo Opportunity
Secluded

FACILITIES
Restrooms
Picnic Tables
Water
Campground

 Wildlife

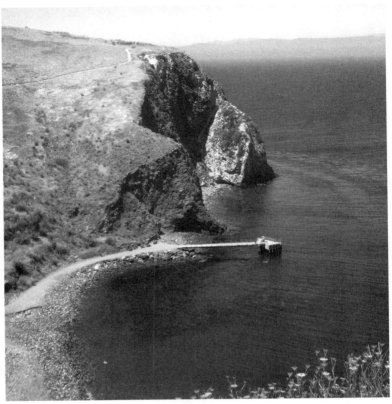

The trail to Cavern Point *carves into the rising bluff above the pier.*

During the short climb, you'll come to a fork ▶2 in the trail, which provides another path to Potato Harbor, located 1.6 miles away. Stay right to reach Cavern Point, which you'll come to at 1.0 mile as you walk along a sheer cliff ▶3 that offers **great views** of the mainland and the eastern portion of the island. The winds can be strong atop the point, so hike carefully along the cliffs. The point gets its name from the marvelous sea caves 310 feet below, which are popular with sea kayakers and home to diverse species of marine life.

M Great Views

Continue clockwise along the loop ▶4 down to the harbor, taking in the view of the mainland and the water along the way. The trail makes its descent to the main access road at 1.6 miles. ▶5 The trail ends at the south end of the campground, ▶6 near the trailhead.

	MILESTONES	
▶1	0.0	Start at the lower Scorpion Campground at the marked trailhead.
▶2	0.3	Stay right at the fork in the trail.
▶3	1.0	Carefully walk up to the cliff's edge, where you can look down to Cavern Point.
▶4	1.2	Continue following the loop clockwise, toward the harbor.
▶5	1.6	Trail descends toward Scorpion Harbor.
▶6	2.0	Trail reaches trailhead, at the south end of the campground.

NOTES

Cave

Hikers will notice a wine-cellar-like cave near the end of the trail. Early island maps show that volcanic caves near Scorpion Ranch were used by islanders to store dairy products prior to refrigeration. Today, big-eared bats often use these caverns for shelter.

Island Foxes

In 2004, the National Park Service released 23 endangered Channel Islands foxes on Santa Rosa and San Miguel islands. Park officials say the foxes were on the brink of extinction at the turn of the 20th century because of golden eagle predation. Some of the foxes were released with radio collars so biologists could monitor their activity. The small, reddish-colored foxes are most often seen roaming about the lower campgrounds in the evening hours.

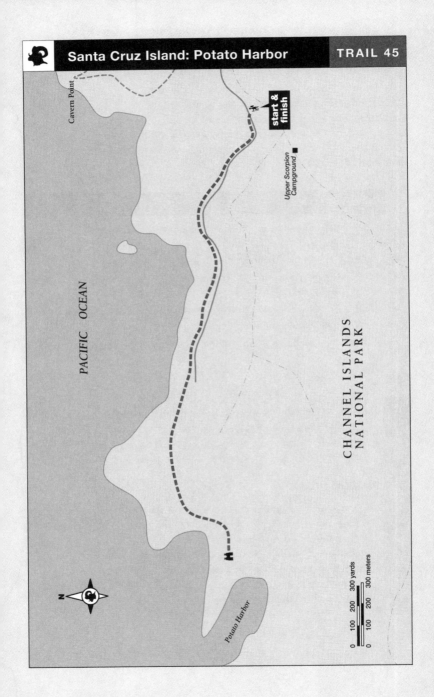

Santa Cruz Island: Potato Harbor TRAIL 45

start & finish

Cavern Point

Upper Scorpion
Campground

PACIFIC OCEAN

CHANNEL ISLANDS
NATIONAL PARK

Potato Harbor

N

0   100   200   300 yards
0   100   200   300 meters

Santa Cruz Island: Potato Harbor

This relatively smooth hike leads to an overlook on the north side of Santa Cruz Island, where you can peer across to the mainland and down to a protected cove called Potato Harbor. The cove is named for its oval shape, which resembles a spud. It's a great perch for wildlife-watchers who want to look down on barking seals and swooping brown pelicans. This trip, like the Cavern Point Trail, is a quick, easy-to-follow hike that's ideal for visitors making a day trip to the Channel Islands.

TRAIL USE
Hike, Run
LENGTH
3.2 miles, 1.5 hours
VERTICAL FEET
±353
DIFFICULTY
– 1 **2** 3 4 5 +
TRAIL TYPE
Out & Back
SURFACE TYPE
Dirt

FEATURES
Child Friendly
Steep
Beach
Birds
Great Views
Photo Opportunity
Secluded

FACILITIES
Restrooms
Picnic Tables
Water
Campground

Best Time

Potato Harbor is picturesque on fog-free afternoons, but if you're hoping to get a clean photo of the cove without any kayakers or boats below, it's best to get to the overlook in the early morning. The overlook is a peaceful spot for a picnic or rest stop away from the screams and splashes near the pier and beach area at Scorpion Anchorage.

Finding the Trail

Island Packers is the authorized charter company for Channel Islands National Park. Reservations can be made at (805) 642-1393. The boat leaves out of Channel Islands Harbor in Ventura and drops passengers off at the Scorpion Harbor Pier on east Santa Cruz.

Take the fire road from the pier past Scorpion Ranch for 0.8 mile to the clearly marked trailhead at the beginning of the second campground. There are no restrooms or water on the hike, although both are available at the campground.

Trail Description

The trail quickly climbs 300 feet in the first 0.7 mile ▶1 and wraps around the west side of the upper **campground**. Keep an eye out for Channel Islands foxes on the lower stretches of the trail near the campground.

The climb is steady and steep, with few trees and even less shade along the way. At 0.9 mile, a trail to Cavern Point branches off the main trail ▶2 to Potato Harbor. The trail begins to flatten out after the first mile, crossing the grassy hillside ▶3 and offering astonishing views of Santa Barbara Channel. The single track continues to follow the bluff around the north end of the Santa Cruz Island coast and on to the lookout above Potato Harbor, ▶4 where the trail ends at 1.6 miles.

Use caution when hiking the later stretches of the trail, as the cliffside shale is very unstable along the bluff trail. Do not hike beyond the overlook to the cove; just return the way you came. You also could return via the Cavern Point Trail, which follows a north bluff trail to Cavern Point and ends near the Scorpion Ranch complex.

⚠ **Camping**

This isolated cove is a favorite spot for California sea lions and harbor seals. The two species rest and breed along Santa Cruz Island's shoreline.

🚶 MILESTONES

▶1	0.0	Start at the trailhead located near the start of the upper campground.
▶2	0.9	Stay straight on the main trail, which branches off to Cavern Point.
▶3	1.3	Hike with caution along the bluff trail, which offers views of he Santa Barbara Channel.
▶4	1.6	Trail ends at the lookout point above Potato Harbor, which can be seen below; return the way you came.

Notice

There is no beach access on this trail, which turns around at the lookout over to Potato Harbor. Hikers are advised not to continue hiking past the lookout point because of the steepness and the unstable shale that comprise the walls of the harbor.

OPTIONS

Other Santa Cruz Island Trails

Aside from the three trails suggested in this book, eastern Santa Cruz Island is home to at least a dozen other maintained trails. A map of the trails is available at the kiosk near the pier at Scorpion Anchorage. Hikers should note that only the trails between Prisoners Harbor and Valley Anchorage are open to the public. No hiking is permitted beyond the national park boundary on land owned by the Nature Conservancy.

From Scorpion Beach, hikers have access to the Scorpion Canyon Loop and Montanon Ridge Trail. The Scorpion Canyon Loop runs past the upper campground and is a 4.5-mile hike up to the interior of the island. The trail eventually ends at a fire road, which meets up with Smugglers Road. Hikers looking for a longer trail can take Smugglers Road down to Smugglers Cove and return to Scorpion Anchorage to complete the loop.

Montanon Ridge is an 8.0-mile trek to the very heart of the islands, with views down to south side of the island, which is rarely seen by the public.

There are three additional trails that begin at Smugglers Cove, including Smugglers Canyon (2.0 miles), Yellowbanks (3.0 miles), and San Pedro Point (4.0 miles). All three are moderate hikes.

From Prisoner's Harbor near the Nature Conservancy boundary, there are five grueling trails: Pelican Bay (4.0 miles), Del Norte Camp (7.0 miles), Del Norte Loop/Navy Road (8.5 miles), Chinese Harbor (15.5 miles), and China Pines (18 miles). The Pelican Bay Trail is open only to hikers who have acquired a permit from the Nature Conservancy or are on a docent-led hike.

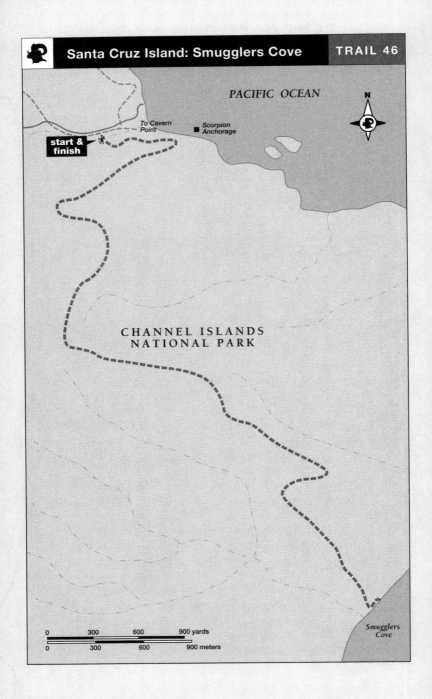

Santa Cruz Island: Smugglers Cove   TRAIL 46

PACIFIC OCEAN

N

To Cavern
Point

Scorpion
Anchorage

start &
finish

CHANNEL ISLANDS
NATIONAL PARK

Smugglers
Cove

0   300   600   900 yards

0   300   600   900 meters

Santa Cruz Island: Smugglers Cove

Smugglers Cove, on the east side of Santa Cruz Island, earned its name from the illicit activities of the sea otter traders and bandits who hid out at the Channel Islands in the late 1700s and early 1800s. Today, it's still a great getaway for sailboats, kayakers, and the hikers willing to make the trek over from Scorpion Beach. The cobblestone beach can be a nice spot for sunbathers when the tide is low and the sandy portion of the beach is unveiled. The warm, clear water is wonderful for wading, snorkeling, or bodysurfing in the small surf. While the water is a bit warmer on this side of the island, the swell is still small, so leave the surfboards at home.

Best Time

Smugglers Cove is beautiful all year. If you're interested in swimming, snorkeling, or bodysurfing, summer is the warmest time to visit. There are no restrooms or water on this side of the island, so prepare accordingly.

Finding the Trail

Island Packers is the authorized charter company for Channel Islands National Park. Reservations can be made at (805) 642-1393. The boat leaves out of Channel Islands Harbor in Ventura and drops passengers off at the Scorpion Harbor Pier on east Santa Cruz. Take the fire road from the pier past Scorpion Ranch for 0.2 mile to the clearly marked trail/fire road to the left (near the windmill).

TRAIL USE
Hike, Run
LENGTH
7.4 miles, 3.5 hours
VERTICAL FEET
±525
DIFFICULTY
– 1 2 3 4 **5** +
TRAIL TYPE
Out & Back
SURFACE TYPE
Dirt

FEATURES
Child Friendly
Steep
Beach
Birds
Great Views
Photo Opportunity
Secluded

FACILITIES
Restrooms
Picnic Tables
Water
Campground

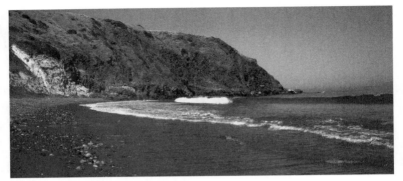

The cobblestone beach *at Smugglers Cove*

Trail Description

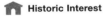

Santa Cruz is the largest island off the West Coast, at 96 square miles and 62,000 acres.

 Historic Interest

Starting at the ranch house, follow the service road, Smugglers Road, to the left past the rusty windmill ▶1 and up to the flats above the canyon. Be prepared to climb a few hundred feet in the first mile. There isn't much elevation gain on the remainder of the hike.

At 1.7 miles, ▶2, the trail meets with the trail to Scorpion Canyon, Montanon Ridge, and the **oil well**. The exploratory well, which was drilled in 1966 by Atlantic Richfield, drew water instead of oil, so no additional oil drilling has ever taken place on the island.

At the 2.0-mile mark, ▶3 you'll see a pile of stones. In the late 1800s, workers on the island cleared the fields of rocks to plant wheat, corn, potatoes, and hay. From here, the trail quickly descends

Wild Boars

NOTES

The skulls and other remains of wild boars may be found in the Smugglers Cove area. Considered a nuisance, this introduced species was common on the island before being eradicated in an effort to protect the native plant species.

to the cobblestone cove at 3.0 miles. ►4 During the descent, the trail passes an olive grove and offers **amazing views** of nearby Anacapa Island.

You'll reach the **cove** at 3.7 miles. ►5 After enjoying the serenity of the cove, return the way you came, pacing yourself over the first mile during the largest elevation gain.

Notice

Fishing is not allowed in the Scorpion State Marine Reserve but is allowed at Smugglers Cove, which is outside the protected marine area. Check current saltwater fishing regulations with the Department of Fish and Game before fishing off the Channel Island coast.

🚶	**MILESTONES**	
►1	0.0	The trail, which follows the service road, starts near the ranch house.
►2	1.7	Stay straight on the main trail.
►3	2.0	Stone piles can be seen off to the right of the trail.
►4	3.0	Trail begins to descend past the olive grove and on to the beach.
►5	3.7	Turn around at the cove and return the way you came.

Santa Cruz Island Camping

OPTIONS

Hike-in camping is permitted at Santa Cruz Island at the upper and lower Scorpion Campgrounds. No fires, however, are allowed in the campground or anywhere on the island. Camping sites do have picnic tables and small storage boxes. Potable water and restrooms are located at each campground. All trash must be packed out, and campers are limited to backpacks that weigh no more than 40 pounds. Reservations can be made with the park by calling (800) 365-2267.

Appendix 1

Top Rated Trails

Chapter 1: Southern Monterey County–Ragged Point
Trail 1: McWay Falls
Trail 3: Limekiln Creek
Trail 5: Salmon Creek Falls

Chapter 2: Northern San Luis Obispo County
Trail 8: San Simeon Point
Trail 11: Elfin Forest
Trail 12: Montaña de Oro Bluff Trail
Trail 13: Coon Creek

Chapter 3: Southern San Luis Obispo County
Trail 21: Bishop Peak
Trail 22: Cerro San Luis
Trail 23: Big Falls

Chapter 4: Santa Barbara County
Trail 30: Gaviota Overlook
Trail 36: Inspiration Point
Trail 37: Seven Falls
Trail 38: Montecito Overlook

Chapter 5: Northern Ventura County–Channel Islands
Trail 41: Matilija Creek
Trail 42: Santa Paula Canyon
Trail 46: Santa Cruz Island: Smugglers Cove

Appendix 2

Public Agencies and Nonprofit Organizations

National Parks

Channel Islands National Park
1901 Spinnaker Dr.
Ventura, CA 93001
(805) 658-5730
www.nps.gov/chis

Los Padres National Forest

Los Padres National Forest Main Office
6755 Hollister Ave., Suite 150
Goleta, CA 93117
(805) 968-6640
www.fs.fed.us/r5/lospadres

Los Padres National Forest Maps
(805) 968-6640
www.fs.fed.us/r5/forestvisitormaps/lospadres
www.nationalforeststore.com

Monterey Ranger District
406 S. Mildred
King City, CA 93930
(831) 385-5434

Mt. Pinos Monterey Ranger District

34580 Lockwood Valley Road
Frazier Park, CA 93225
(661) 245-3731

Ojai Monterey Ranger District

1190 E. Ojai Ave.
Ojai, CA 93023
(805) 646-4348

Santa Barbara Monterey Ranger District

3505 Paradise Road
Santa Barbara, CA 93105
(805) 967-3481

Santa Lucia Monterey Ranger District

1616 N. Carlotti Dr.
Santa Maria, CA 93454
(805) 925-9538

California State Parks

Andrew Molera State Park

Big Sur Station #1
Big Sur, CA 93920
(831) 667-2315

Carpinteria State Beach

Carpinteria, CA 93013
(805) 968-1033

Cayucos State Beach

Cayucos, CA 93430
(805) 781-5930

Chumash Painted Cave State Historic Park

Santa Barbara, CA 93105
(805) 733-3713

El Capitán State Beach

Goleta, CA 93117
(805) 968-1033

El Presidio de Santa Barbara State Historic Park

Santa Barbara, CA 93101
(805) 965-0093

Emma Wood State Beach

Ventura, CA 93001
(805) 968-1033

Estero Bay State Property

Cayucos, CA 93430
(805) 772-7434

Gaviota State Park

Lompoc, CA 93436
(805) 968-1033

Hearst San Simeon State Historical Monument

750 Hearst Castle Road
San Simeon, CA 93452
(805) 927-2020

Julia Pfeiffer Burns State Park

Big Sur Station #1
Big Sur, CA 93920
(831) 667-2315

La Purisima Mission State Historic Park

2295 Purisima Road
Lompoc, CA 93436
(805) 733-3713

Limekiln State Park

Big Sur, CA 93920
(831) 667-2403

Los Osos Oaks State Reserve

Los Osos, CA 93402
(805) 772-7434

McGrath State Beach

Oxnard, CA 93035
(805) 968-1033

Montaña de Oro State Park

Los Osos, CA 93402
(805) 528-0513

Morro Bay State Park

Morro Bay State Park Road
Morro Bay, CA 93442
(805) 772-2560

Morro Strand State Beach

Morro Bay, CA 93442
(805) 772-2560

Oceano Dunes State Vehicle Recreation Area

Oceano, CA 93445
(805) 773-7170

Pfeiffer Big Sur State Park

Big Sur Station #1
Big Sur, CA 93920
(831) 667-2315

Pismo State Beach

555 Pier Ave.
Oceano, CA 93445
(805) 489-1869

Refugio State Beach

10 Refugio Beach Road
Goleta, CA 93117
(805) 968-1033

San Simeon State Park

Van Gordon Creek Road at San Simeon Creek Road
Cambria CA, 93428
(805) 927-2020

William Randolph Hearst Memorial State Beach

750 Hearst Castle Road
San Simeon, CA 93452
(805) 927-2020

County Parks

Monterey County Parks Department

P.O. Box 5249
Salinas, CA 93915
(831) 755-4899
www.co.monterey.ca.us/parks

San Luis Obispo County Parks

1087 Santa Rosa St.
San Luis Obispo, CA 93408
(805) 781-5930
www.slocountyparks.com

Santa Barbara County Parks

Rocky Nook County Park
610 Mission Canyon Road
Santa Barbara, CA 93105
(805) 568-2461
www.sbparks.org

Ventura County Parks Department

800 S. Victoria Ave., L#1030
Ventura, California 93009
(805) 654-3951
www.countyofventura.org

Lake Parks

Lake San Antonio

2610 San Antonio Road
Bradley, CA 93426
(805) 472-2818
www.lakesanantonio.net

Lake Nacimiento

10625 Nacimiento Lake Dr.
Bradley, CA 93426
(805) 238-1056
www.nacimientoresort.com

Santa Margarita Lake

4765 Santa Margarita Lake Road
Santa Margarita, CA 93453
(805) 788-2397
www.slocountyparks.com/activities/santa_margarita.htm

Lopez Lake

4564 Lopez Lake Dr.
Arroyo Grande, CA 93420
(805) 788-2381
www.slocountyparks.com/activities/lopez.htm

Lake Cachuma

HC 59 Hwy. 154
Santa Barbara, CA 93105
(805) 688-4658
www.sbparks.org/DOCS/Cachuma.html

Lake Casitas

11311 Santa Ana Road
Ventura, CA 93001
(805) 649-2233
www.lakecasitas.info

Nonprofit Organizations

Los Padres Chapter of the Sierra Club

P.O. Box 31241
Santa Barbara, CA 93130-1241
(805) 965-9719
www.lospadres.sierraclub.org

Santa Lucia Chapter of the Sierra Club

P.O. Box 15755
San Luis Obispo, CA 93406.
(805) 543-8717
www.santalucia.sierraclub.org

Ventana Chapter of the Sierra Club

P.O. Box 5667
Carmel, CA 93921
(831) 624-8032
www.ventana.sierraclub.org

Appendix 3

Recommended Reading

Dawkins, Gwen, and Dirk Franklin. *Fat Tire Fun: Mountain Biking San Luis Obispo County*. Fat Tire Fun, 1998.

Elliot, Analise. *Hiking & Backpacking Big Sur*. Berkeley, CA: Wilderness Press, 2005.

Krist, John. *50 Best Short Hikes in California's Central Coast*. Berkeley, CA: Wilderness Press, 1998.

Milne, Brian. *Fishing Central California*. Tucson, AZ: No Nonsense Fly Fishing Guidebooks, 2007.

Mohle, Robert. *Adventure Kayaking: Trips from Big Sur to San Diego*. Berkeley, CA: Wilderness Press, 1998.

Sierra Club, Santa Lucia Chapter. *Sierra Club San Luis Obispo County Trail Guide*, 1989.

Stienstra, Tom, and Ann Marie Brown. *California Hiking*. Emeryville, CA: Avalon Travel Publishing, 2005.

Stob, Ron. *Exploring San Luis Obispo County*. San Luis Obispo, CA: Central Coast Press, 1998.

Stone, Robert. *Day Hikes on the California Central Coast*. Pismo Beach, CA: Day Hike Books, Inc., 2001.

Index

Author

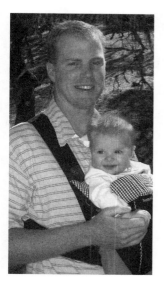

Brian Milne

A California native, Brian Milne is an avid outdoorsman and writer who grew up hiking, mountain biking, kayaking, and fishing in Central California. Milne earned his bachelors degree in journalism at California Polytechnic State University and is an award-winning senior reporter for *The Tribune* newspaper in San Luis Obispo, California. He also contributes regularly to outdoors magazines and websites. His first guidebook, *Fishing Central California*, was published by No Nonsense Fly Fishing Guidebooks in 2007. Milne enjoys the outdoors with his wife, Aja, and with his daughter, Payton, to whom this guide is dedicated.

More **TOP TRAILS**™ from **WILDERNESS PRESS**

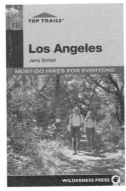

ISBN 0-89997-347-7

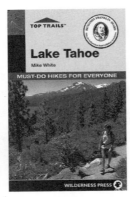

ISBN 978-0-89997-349-4

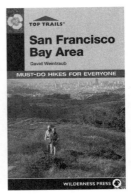

ISBN 0-89997-348-5

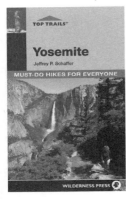

ISBN 978-0-89997-425-5

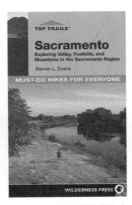

ISBN 978-0-89997-381-4

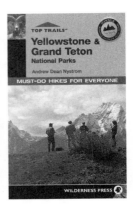

ISBN 978-0-89997-368-5

For ordering information, contact your local bookseller
or **Wilderness Press, www.wildernesspress.com**